Conquer Your Balance Disorder

Revised Edition

Everything you need to know about your balance
disorder and how to "fix" it

Andrew Goldbaum

ISBN-10: 1543221505

ISBN-13: 978-1543221503

Dedication:

To my mom and dad; they deserve much more than I can ever give…

Table of Contents

WARNING

Dizziness may be an indicator of a serious medical condition. These conditions may include but are not limited to: Stroke, blood clot, circulatory problem, heart attack, high or low blood pressure, brain tumor, Lyme disease or other serious disease or condition.

IF YOU ARE CURRENTLY EXPERIENCING DIZZINESS SEEK IMMEDIATE MEDICAL ATTENTION

Only after a doctor determines that your condition is not serious or life threatening should you continue reading this book!

DISCLAIMER

I am not a doctor, nutritionist or healthcare professional. In addition, being human, I may have made mistakes or omissions. Consult your doctor before considering any exercise, treatment, supplement, dietary change or anything else suggested in this book.

Unfortunately, although I sincerely hope it does, I can't guarantee that this book will help with your dizziness, balance, tinnitus or any other conditions discussed in this book. In fact, what helped me may be extremely harmful to you or may even make your condition worse. This is why I strongly recommend consulting your doctor before trying or emulating anything in this book!

Preface

When I had my first balance/dizziness attack, I thought I was going to die. I felt so profoundly ill I didn't even realize I was dizzy. I was driven to the hospital emergency room where any serious medical condition was ruled out and I was diagnosed with vertigo. Later after many such attacks, visits to specialists and sophisticated testing, I realized that my vertigo now diagnosed as Meniere's disease was here to stay. There was apparently no doctor, pill, or therapy that would be able to help my condition. No one could tell me its cause or why I was the lucky one who got it. My life was day after day of suffering, wondering if I would be able to drive to work, get through an entire day, or drive home.

I was single and tried my best to have a normal social life, but attacks while I was out ended that. I saw my family very little. The noise of family gatherings only seemed to aggravate my condition. Everywhere I went, I seemed to be racing against an invisible clock. Would I be able to finish my food shopping, banking or visit to the department store before the next attack hit? Would I be able to drive home and reach the safe haven of my couch in time? Would I be able to sleep peacefully or be awakened by recurring dreams of riding on various amusement park rides?

I suffered from severe Meniere's disease for over three years until by luck I was referred to a nutritionist with a background in biochemistry. He was able to diagnose the cause of my problem and suggest a treatment consisting of a diet and supplements that ultimately reduced my symptoms to practically zero within a few months. By reading this book and learning from my experience, you should be able to work with your own doctor or healthcare professional to reduce your symptoms and have a normal life again.

The relationship among diet, biochemistry and balance disorders seems to be almost unknown to medical science. Many doctors still seem to believe that most balance disorders are psychological and caused by stress and will likely suggest seeing a psychologist. I seem to be the only person suggesting this alternative solution to overcoming balance problems. From my own experience and the hundreds emails I have received from a balance disorder website that I had operated for over a decade, I know my concept is relevant for many people[1]. It is my hope that by using my diet and supplement regimen as a model and with help from your doctor, that you can reduce your symptoms as significantly as I did and have a life again[2].

---

[1] This book provides significantly expanded, updated, and corrected content from my website which I operated for over 10 years.

[2] Although my diet and supplement regimen consists of over the counter vitamins and supplements and my diet is simple, since everyone is different, it may actually be harmful for you. Consult your doctor before trying anything in this book.

Preface Part 2

In January 2017 it struck again. When I awoke one morning I felt like I was spinning faster than could be possible in real life. I sat up in bed and after a twenty second eternity, the spinning subsided. Lying down again restarted the spinning. I knew at once I had Benign Paroxysmal Positional Vertigo (BPPV) which is different from Meniere's disease and is much more likely to be "curable". It occurred when I tilted my head back or to the right or to a lesser extent down.

I decided to go to an Ear, Nose and Throat (ENT) doctor to confirm my self-diagnosis and pick up some medication that would help reduce my symptoms. As is typical, that's all they could do for me. They also gave me an informational pamphlet on what causes dizziness.

At home, I tried to do the Epley Maneuver as described later in this book. I became so dizzy during the attempt that I couldn't even complete the first step. I decided to see a second ENT more experienced with balance disorders.

The second ENT was more helpful as she gave me a more useful pamphlet. It was for a local Physical Therapy center that had a therapist very experienced with balance disorders which is a rarity. To make a short story even shorter, the therapist carefully guided me through the Epley maneuver, holding my head and telling me when I would feel dizzy and when it would subside. The first time was horrible and felt like I was thrown off a cliff, but I didn't get dizzy the second time. This meant it worked, no more BPPV, at least until about 4AM when it hit again. This time I was able to do the Epley Maneuver myself while still in bed since the BPPV was less severe. I have not had a reoccurrence since.

It was after this second bout of dizziness from BPPV that I decided to update this book. It contains updated information, corrections and a more detailed section on BPPV. It's also less expensive because it's printed in black and white instead of color. I sincerely hope it helps you!

HELP ME NOW!!

If you purchased this book because you are suffering from a balance problem and want quick relief, try the suggestions below. It's very likely that these suggestions will help you feel somewhat better in just a day or two.

<u>Remember - Check with your doctor before trying these suggestions!</u>

1. Go on a low salt diet of 1,000-1,200 mg per day. Excess salt makes you retain water and may affect your inner ear. Keeping your sodium and hydration level very constant will help. See the diet chapter (14) of this book.

2. Drink at least eight, 8 oz. glasses of water per day. Drink more during hot weather and if you exercise. A constant level of hydration will help your balance problem.

3. Avoid <u>all</u> caffeine. No caffeinated coffee, tea, energy drinks, energy shots, caffeine inhalers or even chocolate. Decaffeinated coffee and tea contains some caffeine so try to avoid these as well.

4. Avoid all alcohol (including wine). In addition to affecting your hydration level, alcohol adversely affects balance. The sulfite preservatives in many wines may also cause additional problems.

5. If your doctor agrees, take non-drowsy anti-histamine such as Claritin®.

6. Avoid all sugar (sucrose). This sounds impossible, but it can be done. Sugar causes an adrenalin release that may trigger balance attacks.

7. Avoid stimulants such as Ginkgo Biloba, energy drinks and energy boosters. Some herbal supplements are stimulants that may adversely affect your balance.

8. Avoid stress. Keep as relaxed as possible. I know it's not easy to do.

9. Avoid eating in restaurants. Most restaurant food (especially fast food) is very high in sodium and may contain monosodium glutamate (MSG) which may act as a stimulant and adversely affect balance. Avoid spicy foods.

10. Use a HEPA air filter and stay indoors as much as possible during hay fever season. This will help reduce the particles you inhale which may cause allergy symptoms. Use a humidifier if it's very dry.

11. No smoking!

12. If you are dizzy only when your head is in specific positions you may have BPPV. Find a therapy center that can perform the Epley maneuver.

13. Do not use any "recreational drugs". None have been shown to help balance disorders and getting proper treatment for your balance disorder while in prison is very unlikely.

Chapter 1: Life Before, During and After (My Balance Attack)

Before:

I had a normal life like (most) any other 29 year old.

During:

I was sitting at my desk on a typical workday in May 1993 when suddenly I was overwhelmed with nausea. I had no chest pain but thought I was having a heart attack. I was confused, had trouble breathing, and could hardly walk. I thought I was going to die.

After taking my pulse and realizing my heart was still beating regularly (although rapidly), a friend drove me to the emergency room. Luckily, my family doctor was on call. After a preliminary check-up which included an Electrocardiogram (ECG or EKG) and blood test, ruled out anything immediately life threatening, my doctor held up his pen and told me to look at the tip. After a few seconds he said you have Vertigo. My eyes were moving rapidly from side to side (called Nystagmus) indicating a dizzy patient. At the time I felt so disoriented and nauseous, I didn't even realize I was dizzy.

After:

After this initial (balance/dizziness attack) episode, I spent the next three days in bed, incapacitated and heavily medicated on Antivert®. Antivert® is one of the medications available that (somewhat) relieves the symptoms of a balance disorder. When I was finally able to get out of bed, I still needed to take the medication so I could function in my everyday life. I was constantly dizzy to varying degrees and usually had a few severe balance attacks daily. I had to take Antivert® for a while even though it made me absolutely exhausted. It made me so tired that I finally resolved only to take it when I had attacks, not just to relieve my continual day to day dizziness. When attacks did occur, they were incapacitating for the few minutes to an hour or so in which they lasted. During these attacks I felt nausea and dizziness so severe that I hoped I would "pass out", but I never did. Despite my ceaseless suffering, I continued to go to work and attend a graduate program at a local college. The attacks forced me to leave work or class early on many occasions. Sometimes I was just too dizzy to go at all. I had a constant fear that an attack would incapacitate me without notice causing an embarrassing scene at work, school or in public.

After I settled into the pattern of dealing with Meniere's disease on a daily basis, I began to take stock of myself. I realized that I had lost much of my coordination, had concentration problems, panic attacks and memory trouble as well as a reduced appetite. I frequently had various degrees of ringing in one or both ears. Many times while walking I needed to touch a wall for support. Sometimes, for a brief second it would feel like the floor dropped out from under me. Darkened rooms were nearly impossible for me to navigate without touching walls and furniture as if I were blind. My social life disappeared.

I tried to keep fit by exercising at home. Weight lifting made me very dizzy during and immediately after the activity. The stair stepper machine also made me dizzy during and immediately after, especially when I stepped off the machine, but I actually felt very good about an hour later. This "good" feeling would last a few hours so I tried to make using it routine, as it was usually the only relief I could count on.

Another activity that usually made me feel somewhat better was driving a car. This is because my interaction with the steering wheel and the car's subsequent movement; linked my muscles', visual and inner ear's perception of motion. It's the disagreement of perceived motion among your muscles, eyes and ears that cause dizziness. I used to drive to my destination and then feel terrible when I would get out of the car. Being a passenger in a car was a nauseating experience whether the car was a smooth driving Cadillac or a bumpy SUV. Although the bumpier the ride, the worse I felt. Before Meniere's disease I could read in a car while a passenger, an activity that even makes many "normal" people feel sick. After Meniere's, this was impossible.

Frequently, my suffering would even continue while I was sleeping. Often I would have dreams that involved spinning such as riding a carousel, rolling down a hill, being in a car going around a continuous tight curve, etc., making me nauseous even while sleeping. Occasionally the nausea would be so bad it would actually wake me up in the middle of the night. Sometimes I had to get out of bed to take Antivert® to be able to get back to sleep.

Today:

After making a substantial recovery from my balance disorder and my recent BPPV episode, I feel fine. I was even a student pilot for a while, completing about 80 hours of flight training mostly in a Cessna 172. This is a testament to how substantially my condition improved.

After remaining on my diet and supplement program for many years, I slowly began to cheat. When I feel symptoms start to return, such as feeling foggy, having my ears start ringing a bit or becoming a little dizzy, I adhere to my regimen more strictly. The fact that my balance problem begins to return when I cheat (too much) confirms at least for me that my regimen is effective. Let's face it; it's not easy eating the same foods and taking the same supplements for over two decades. My cheating mostly consists of eating dark chocolate, a couple of extra slices of bread, the occasional brownie, cookies and Chinese food. When I did adhere strictly to the diet I was never hungry and rarely had an urge to cheat. However, chocolate and sugar are addictive (literally), so it takes at least one week of not eating them to stop any cravings. The biggest change is that I take very few supplements; just once a day instead of many pills three times a day as originally "prescribed". I originally reduced my supplements to twice a day due to gastric reflux I was experiencing. I've since resolved this with 20 mg of Omeprazole® (antacid) per day which is available by prescription. Zegerid OTC® is available over the counter with the same ingredient but it contains quite a bit of Sodium Bicarbonate. Sodium Bicarbonate becomes Sodium when digested which is not good for your health in general and is terrible for Meniere's sufferers. I have reduced my supplements to the bare minimum that is effective after an episode in which some were actually contaminated with steroids[3].

By not eating dairy products for so many years as per my Meniere's diet, I have become lactose intolerant and can't tolerate dairy products. I do take Lactaid® on occasion when I can't be sure if there is milk in what I'm eating and have no other dietary option available.

My blood tests while on this regimen have always been excellent although sometimes borderline high on sugar. My cardiologist has always been amazed by my extremely low cholesterol level and frequently asks me how I do it.

---

[3] See chapter 24, Postscript

Chapter 2: What is Meniere's Disease?

Meniere's disease is a balance disorder named after the French Doctor who first identified it in the 1860's. Basically the disease has the effect of making the sufferer dizzy and possibly nauseous for periods ranging from a few minutes to several hours. Meniere's disease can also cause a ringing in the ears called Tinnitus (pronounced "tin-eye-tus"). The ringing can be anywhere from barely audible to deafeningly loud and be a serious problem in itself. The amount of dizziness the sufferer feels can range from mild to incapacitating. Unfortunately, no one knows for sure exactly what causes the disease. It is generally agreed that Meniere's symptoms are caused by the failure of a mysterious fluid regulation system that allows too much fluid into the semi-circular canals of the balance (or vestibular) organ located in the inner ear. This extra fluid apparently has an effect on the hair cells in the semi-circular canals causing a balance problem. Some believe that this change in fluid level alters the pressure within the inner ear and it is this pressure that causes the balance problem. The medical community seems to have settled on too much fluid being the issue which justifies (to them and their patients) some of the surgical treatments they offer.

I have seen many statistics of how many people have Meniere's disease. The one that is most believable is that there are over five million people in the United States and 23 million worldwide that have it. Although Meniere's disease is not fatal, sometimes the symptoms are so severe that sufferers are afraid it might be. Many otherwise completely healthy people feel that their lives are over

13

because they live in constant fear of balance attacks, losing their jobs, their social life, have trouble raising their children, or not being as active as they want to be. This bleak outlook is common for the first few months after the onset of the disease. Many people who get Meniere's disease become extremely depressed.

Unfortunately, there is no cure for Meniere's disease. However, many people have achieved various degrees of relief for themselves by taking various medications, going on a low salt diet, participating in vestibular therapy or having drastic and not so drastic surgeries done. Still there is no permanent cure.

Chapter 3: See a Doctor Immediately!!!

The following is so important it gets its own chapter in large print:

There are a variety of tests doctors can use to diagnose Meniere's disease and it's <u>extremely important</u> that they be done as soon as symptoms occur. These tests can rule out more serious conditions that may be causing the loss of balance including but <u>not</u> limited to: a tumor, blood clot, Lyme disease, high or low blood pressure, growth on the auditory nerve or a serious circulatory problem within the brain. Chances are very good that nothing life threatening is wrong, but don't take a chance. **See a doctor immediately!**

Chapter 4: Medical Testing (Overview)

I went to many doctors during the three years I suffered from Meniere's disease. At first, I saw doctors to confirm that my symptoms were not caused by anything serious or life threatening. I had X-rays, a computed tomography (CT or "Cat") scan, Magnetic resonance imaging (MRI), and neurological and audiology tests to rule out the potentially more serious causes of my disorder. After the doctors were satisfied that my condition was not life threatening, I went to several ear, nose and throat (ENT) doctors and neurologists specializing in balance disorders to find a "cure". Each specialist ran me through tests to discover the extent of my disorder. Some tests like the Electronystagmography (ENG) and hearing tests were repeated several times by different doctors who didn't want to rely on previous results. I even saw a specialist who worked with NASA designing balance experiments for space shuttle astronauts. The doctors I went to, the tests they performed, and the reason they performed them are listed below.

Medical Testing		
Doctor	**Test**	**Reason**
Internist	Eye movement test.	Initial diagnosis of vertigo. Rapid left and right eye movement (nystagmus) is a classic indicator of a balance problem.
Neurologist	Checked the movement and sensation in my, head, neck, limbs and eyes.	Checked for nervous system damage that may be caused by a growth in the brain. This test was done prior to taking any X-rays or other imaging.
	Checked hearing and the noises produced by the bones of the inner ear.	Checked for possible growth on inner ear canal or auditory nerve.
Audiologist	Complete hearing test.	Checked for hearing loss which occurs many times with a balance disorder.
Ear, Nose, Throat (ENT)	Examined my ears, nose and throat.	Checked for ear damage, sinus abnormality/ infection and presence of past or existing virus that may have caused damage to my balance organ.
	X-ray and CT scan of sinus, inner ear area.	Checked for abnormal growths in the inner ear and sinus area.

Doctor	Test	Reason
Balance Specialist Neurologist	MRI of brain.	Checked for any growths in the brain.
	Falling test: With one foot directly in front of the other and my eyes closed, checked in which direction I would tend to fall.	You tend to fall towards the side in which the damage to the vestibular organ occurred. Obviously the doctor did not let me actually fall.
	Straight line walking test. With my eyes open then closed, I walked normally and then lifted my knees up as if I were marching.	Checked to see if my gait (or stride) was affected by the disorder and confirmed the side of the damage. You tend to "march" to the side of damage when your eyes are closed.
	Electronystagmography (ENG)/ Caloric Balance test	Checked to see the extent of the damage done to the vestibular organ.
	Rotating chair test	More accurate check to see the extent of the damage done to the vestibular organ.

Doctor	Test	Reason
Balance Specialist (ENT)	Checked for ear damage	Checked for ear damage, sinus abnormality/ infection and presence of past or existing virus that may have caused damage.
Allergist	Scratch test and Immunoglobulin/ Rast blood test.	Attempted to discover an immune/ allergic cause for my disorder.

Chapter 5: Medical Testing (Detail)

The following provides a more detailed explanation of the sophisticated testing I had done:

Electronystagmography (ENG) Balance Test:

The Electronystagmography (ENG) Balance test is a diabolical test used to determine the extent of damage to the balance system by making you dizzy. It is also used to determine if the balance problem is caused by your brain or inner ear. Several electrodes are placed on the forehead and (possibly) face to monitor the tiny electrical currents generated by your eyes when they look right or left. A charge difference between parts of your eye (called corneal-retinal potential) creates an electrical signal. When you look right a very small positive electrical current is generated. A very small negative current is generated when you look left. The object of the test is to make you dizzy, which causes your eyes to move rapidly from left to right or right to left. This eye movement is measured by graphing the small electrical currents picked up by the electrodes on your forehead using a computer. The speed in which your eyes move is a measure of how dizzy you are. Videonystagmography (VNG) is identical to an ENG, but uses an infrared camera to track eye movement instead of electrodes.

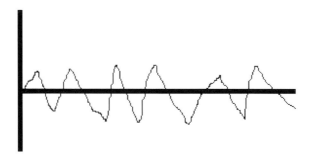

Illustration: Simulated ENG Eye Motion Plot

Here's the diabolical (Caloric) part of the test. In order to make you dizzy (or much dizzier than you currently are) so that the measurements can be made, a special apparatus very much like an old fashioned headphone or shooting earmuff is placed over the ears. The "earmuff" has a plastic tube in the center that partially inserts into your ear canal. Cold water from the apparatus is allowed to continuously flow through this tube, hitting your ear drum with the deafening sound of a raging river. After bouncing off your ear drum, the water flowing out of your ear canal is collected in the earmuff cup where another plastic tube allows the water to drain into a bucket. Because the test is performed while you are lying down and the earmuff fit around your ear isn't perfect, water also tends to leak onto your shirt, your hair, the table, floor, etc. The cold water flowing against your ear drum causes your inner ear to be cool on the water flow side and warmer on the other. This induces convection current (or a circular flow) of the balance fluid in your inner ear in one direction and makes you feel like you're spinning to the right (for example). The spinning feeling quickly increases until its

21

peak. This makes you feel anywhere from a little to unbelievably dizzy and can be very unpleasant.

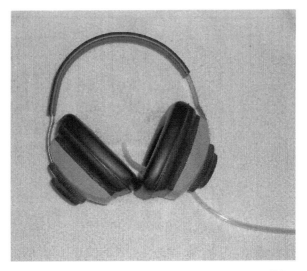

Illustration: Typical Caloric Water Test "Earmuffs"

After the measurements are made, the water is shut off and you gradually return to "normal". The test is then repeated on the same ear with warm water, causing you to "spin" in the other direction. The whole process is repeated with your other ear.

This test can also be performed using a device that shoots a deafening, continuous blast of warm or cold air into your ear canal. This method is just as nauseating, but much less messy. It is used less often because the water test produces better results and does not have any expensive mechanical or electrical parts. The Caloric water test just requires two buckets, some fish tank tubing, a modified earmuff and some caulking to seal the tubing to the earmuffs. The devices I encountered (even the one at a very prestigious hospital) look very much "homemade".

Rotating Chair Test:

The rotating chair balance test is much more sophisticated and sensitive than the Electronystagmography (ENG) Balance test, but is also used to determine the extent of damage to the balance system by making you dizzy. In this test, you sit in a motorized chair in a small circular booth (usually) with black and white vertical stripes painted on the wall. The chair can be spun left or right with very precisely controlled acceleration and speed. The object of the test is to make you dizzy, which causes your eyes to move rapidly from left to right or right to left. Your eye movements are precisely tracked by an infrared video camera (instead of electrodes) that's mounted to special glasses or a holder similar to a welder's mask that attaches to your head. The output of the camera is connected to a computer that charts your eye movement. There are many detailed aspects to this test, but essentially the chair spins you in one direction in complete darkness for several minutes. When the chair is started spinning, there is an initial jolt to the right or left. You feel very dizzy at first, but then as your balance organs adjust to the movement, you feel like you're slowing down and then eventually standing still even though you're still spinning at a constant rate. This is because your balance organ can only sense acceleration and since the chair is moving at a constant speed (soon after the initial jolt), there is none. Just when you get used to the calm sensation of spinning without feeling anything (except a breeze), the chair is suddenly stopped. Now much to your surprise, you feel like you're spinning again (in the opposite direction) and get very dizzy even though the chair is now motionless. The dizziness causes your eyes to move rapidly back and forth. Your eye movement is monitored by the infrared camera system until you return to normal. The test is then performed again in the other direction.

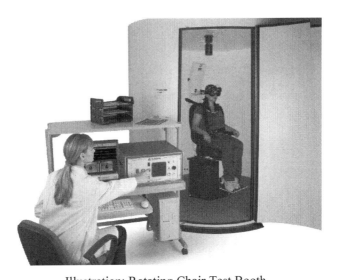

Illustration: Rotating Chair Test Booth
(The image is furnished by Micromedical Technologies, 10 Kemp Drive, Chatham, IL 62629)

Allergy Scratch Test:

The scratch test is commonly used by allergists to determine what compounds a person might be allergic to. By asking you a series of questions about your lifestyle and what you eat, the doctor identifies 20 to 30 compounds that you come into contact with on a daily basis to which you might be allergic (e.g. tree pollen, milk, dust, a cat, etc.). The allergist has dozens of tiny vials at his disposal. Each vial contains a sterile liquid with a suspension of a compound you will be tested with. The compounds include: dog dander, grass pollen, milk protein, etc. A single drop of each compound (including two control compounds) is placed along the inside of your forearm while it lies on a table palm up. A number is marked on your arm in pen near each drop to identify the compound from the list created by the doctor. Sometimes the test is done on the patient's back if many more compounds are to be tested. A small pin is used to scratch the surface of the skin through each drop of liquid. While this doesn't hurt, it allows the liquid from each individual drop to come into contact with fresh skin. After a few minutes, the drops of liquid are removed and the arm is observed for bumps. The bigger the bump caused by a particular compound, the more allergic you are to it. One control compound will always cause a bump while the other will never cause a bump. This allows a doctor to make sure that the test was effective. If it is determined that you do have an allergy to one or more compounds, avoiding them or receiving allergy shots may help your balance disorder.

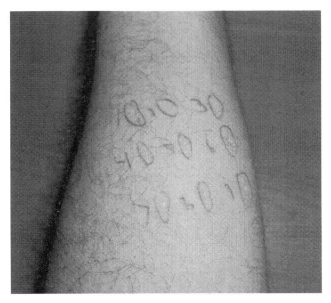

Illustration: Typical Scratch Test markings with drops of various compounds

RAST (RadioAllergoSorbent Test) Blood Test:

If the scratch test fails to indicate that any allergies are present, a much more sensitive Immunoglobulin/ RAST test may be used. This sophisticated test involves drawing several tubes of blood which are sent to a test lab. This test can be very expensive depending on how many potential allergens you are being tested for. This test is extremely sensitive and will let you know for certain if you are at all allergic to any of the compounds you are being tested for. Generally the RAST tests for many more compounds than the scratch test.

My Test Results:

At this point, my medical results indicated that I was completely normal in every way, except for a loss of balance and a minor hearing loss in my right ear. The tests failed to detect any allergies whatsoever. Despite the sophistication and expense of all these tests and the nausea and hardship I endured being subjected to them, they did not determine the cause of my balance disorder nor offer any potential cure.

Chapter 6: How Balance Works

Each (inner) ear, in addition to having all the mechanisms required for hearing, contains a tiny balance organ that's about the size of a quarter. This organ consists of three semi-circular canals or hollow tubes connected to the vestibule.

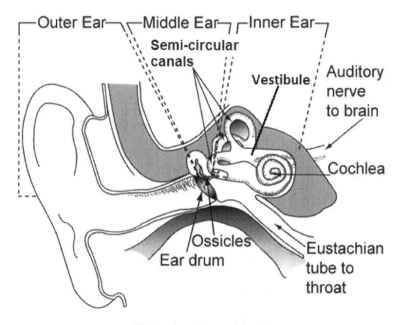

Illustration: Parts of the Ear

(Courtesy weboflife.nasa.gov)

Each semi-circular canal detects when your head undergoes one of three directions of motion called, "pitch", "roll", and "yaw". Yaw motion is when you move your head side to side saying "No". Pitch motion is when you nod you head up and down saying "Yes". Roll motion is when your head tilts from side to side, like when you're starting to fall asleep

27

while sitting upright. These terms are frequently used to describe the motion of an aircraft. In addition, the canals can also detect up and down acceleration like is present in an elevator.

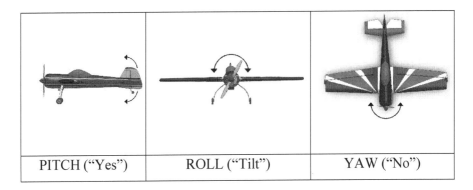

| PITCH ("Yes") | ROLL ("Tilt") | YAW ("No") |

Illustration: Definition of Pitch, Roll and Yaw Motion
(Airplane Courtesy Alexey Yukish)

Each semi-circular tube is filled with a liquid called endolymph. At the bottom of the semi-circular canal is the Ampulla, which contains the structures (saccule and utricle) that detect acceleration (motion) via the Crista. The Crista is composed of hair cells (connected to the balance nerves), the Otolithic membrane which is a gelatin like interface between the hair cells, and the Otoliths (which are tiny sand like grains of calcium carbonate) that are stuck to the top. When your head is moved (accelerated), it causes the Crista to bend due to the brief flow of the endolymph and the mass of the Otoliths. This bending sends signals from the Crista's nerve cells to the brain, which is interpreted as the direction of acceleration of the movement of your head. Your inner ear only detects acceleration, not continuous motion. This is why even though the Rotating chair (described above) is continuously spinning you feel like you are not moving. You can only feel when spinning starts and stops. Likewise when you're on a train or an elevator, you do not feel that you are moving unless it accelerates or decelerates. This is because the Crista only bends during acceleration or deceleration. It's really quite an amazing system.

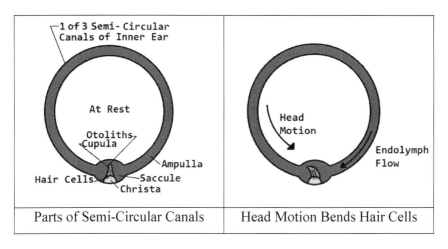

| Parts of Semi-Circular Canals | Head Motion Bends Hair Cells |

Illustration: How the Inner Ear's Semi-circular Canal Works

The reason you feel dizzy when you have a balance disorder is that there is a conflict that occurs among signals from your right inner ear, your left inner ear, your vision, and to some extent your body's awareness of muscle position. For example, your damaged right inner ear may be sending false signals to your brain that your head is being turned to the right. Your left inner ear and vision will be sending signals to your brain that you are not turning. This conflict is interpreted by your brain as dizziness. Many people experience this same dizzying conflict when they are reading while driving (hopefully only as a passenger). The balance organ in each ear sends signals to the brain as they accelerate, turn, bump up and down, etc. The signals from the eyes, because they are focused on the book, are indicating that very little or no motion is occurring. This conflict in signals causes dizziness in most people.

Chapter 7: Balance Attack Causes

It's been my experience that most people who develop balance disorders have an attack out of the blue without any discernable cause just as I had. However if there was a cause it might include becoming dizzy after an auto accident or fall (even weeks afterward), having an attack while sick with a cold, flu or ear infection, and in rare cases being effected by a loud noise or explosion. A balance disorder might also be caused by sudden acceleration or deceleration, by a change in pressure outside the ear during a flight or a mountain drive, while swimming or even while chewing. It is also possible to have an attack while on antibiotics. There are a few common physical causes of balance problems. They are:

- Displaced "Otoconia". Otoconia are small crystals of calcium carbonate that become detached from the balance mechanism and float in the endolymph fluid within the inner ear. They are a normal part of the balance system when attached, but can cause problems if they are in the wrong location in the inner ear. The condition they cause is called Benign Paroxysmal Positional Vertigo (BPPV) or Benign Positional Vertigo (BPV). It's estimated that this is the cause of 20% of balance disorders. Chapter 21 discusses BPPV. With BPPV, certain head positions such as leaning back can cause mild to profound dizziness.

- Vasovagal response. The Vasovagal nerve travels from the base of the brainstem down the neck, to the stomach area and the intestines.

A Vasovagal response occurs when the nerve is irritated or stimulated and triggers a primitive survival response built into your nervous system. It causes slowing of heart and breathing and a drop in blood pressure. It can also cause headache, fainting as well as dizziness. The nerve can be triggered by stress, stomach virus or acid reflux.

- Blood flow (circulatory) causes. Problems with blood circulation in the brain or inner ear including high or low blood pressure can cause dizziness. This is more common in older adults.

- Inner ear fluid problems. A very common type of damage done to the inner ear is to the endolymph fluid regulation system discussed earlier. The inner ear's balance mechanism utilizes endolymph fluid for its operation. Dizziness or a balance attacks occur when there is a problem with the system regulating the amount of endolymph. It's known that too much endolymph causes a balance problem. It's also likely that pressure changes in the inner ear do as well. This balance problem is classified as Meniere's disease. With Meniere's disease you are usually dizzy no matter the position of your head although some positions can be worse than others.

Chapter 8: One Time and Recurring Balance Attacks

There are generally three types of events that cause balance problems. They are one time or single event attacks, multiple event attacks and head movement if the person has BPPV. A single event balance attack may be caused by damage to the inner ear inflicted by a head injury, virus, ear infection or even an extremely loud noise. When a balance attack is caused in this way, there is a one time "attack" of dizziness (that may last from minutes to days) due to damage to the inner ear. While the inner ear that was damaged may heal somewhat, the majority of the recovery happens because the brain compensates for the damage by adjusting how it interprets signals from the other (hopefully) undamaged inner ear. Gradually, over a period from days to a few months, the dizziness subsides and balance returns to near normal.

Multiple event balance attacks are balance attacks that reoccur periodically. They can reoccur at any time from a few minutes to several months apart with a few days to few weeks being the most common interval. The attacks can occur without warning or be preceded by ringing or a feeling of ear pressure and range in severity from mild to incapacitating. After each attack, the dizziness gradually subsides as the actual cause of the attack dissipates and the brain and body compensate for the new state of balance signals. Unfortunately, before balance returns to (near) normal, another attack occurs and not only interrupts the recovery process, but starts it from the beginning again. This cycle of recurring attacks is common to Meniere's suffers.

Dizziness that does not substantially improve over time, gets better then worse or just gets worse is most likely an indication that damage to the inner ear is continuing to occur and that the cause of the balance attack was probably not a onetime event such as an ear infection. This cycle of continuous or periodic inner ear damage and compensation can make the sufferer feel miserable for years and is also typical of Meniere's disease.

Each time damage (or balance loss) occurs to one balance organ (on the right side for example), the brain compensates by "lowering" the sensitivity of the other (left side) organ. Theoretically, if you start off with a balance "level" of 100 and 10% (which is an exaggerated number) is lost on average each time damage occurs, your level will change as shown: 100, 90, 81, 73, 66, 60, etc. During the first balance loss, your brain has to compensate for a 10 point balance drop, which is the worst. The second time the loss occurs your brain has to compensate for a 9 point drop. Although this is terrible, it isn't as bad as the first occurrence. With each 10% loss in balance, your brain has less and less to compensate for; therefore each time a loss occurs it can be less severe. Of course this doesn't hold true if you lose 5% the first time and 8% the second, etc. This may be why some people's balance problem appears to "burn itself out" after a few years. They just get to a point where the amount of damage that is periodically occurring to the balance center is negligible compared to the small amount of "balance" that remains.

Chapter 9: Doctors and Cures

Most doctors know very little about balance disorders; probably because their exposure to them is so limited unlike the seasonal flu, latest stomach virus or cold going around, etc. Once your doctor has decided your aren't in immediate danger from your balance problem, he will likely prescribe Antivert® or something similar in the short term. He may also prescribe Xanax® or alike to help you reduce your anxiety.

Unfortunately, even a specialist in balance disorders (such as my NASA experienced doctor) will not have much more to offer. After all the testing (described above) is completed and your doctor is certain your balance disorder is not caused by anything serious, he will likely just suggest a more modern version of Antivert®, a low salt diet, possibly a diuretic and discuss some surgical options. There are other treatment options available that are discussed below that may provide some relief.

Medications

Antihistamine:

Taking a specialized antihistamine such as Antivert® (or the generic version, Meclizine®) is pretty much the only option when it comes to quickly reducing the symptoms of a balance or dizziness attack. Essentially these antihistamines act to desensitize your brain to the troublesome nerve impulses being transmitted to it by your defective inner ear, relieving some of the nausea and dizziness symptoms. The problem is that the antihistamines prescribed for balance disorders are able to permeate the membrane that surrounds your brain, making you anywhere from a little tired to nearly unconscious. Over time you do get somewhat used to these medications and are less affected by their sleep inducing properties. An antihistamine may also have the added benefit of reducing the effect of histamine on your inner ear which may also help you feel better.

The two antihistamine medications I was prescribed were Meclizine (a.k.a Antivert®) and Promethazine. Promethazine made me much less tired than Antivert®, but it still made me so tired that I tried to take only half a pill and only when I had dizziness attacks. A non-drowsy antihistamine such as Claritin® may also be helpful and make you feel less dizzy as it will help clear the sinuses.

Diuretic:

One medication that can be somewhat effective for Meniere's sufferers is a diuretic. It's likely the next thing after Antivert® your doctor will ask you to try to help reduce your symptoms. It's used to remove salt (sodium) from the body by causing you to urinate (embarrassingly) more frequently. Too much salt causes the body to retain fluids, supposedly elevating the fluid level or pressure in the inner ear and increasing Meniere's symptoms. Reducing the sodium level in your body is best done by a strict low salt diet around 1,000-1,200 mg a day, with sodium intake distributed as evenly as possible over the course of the day. However sodium reduction can often be helped along with a diuretic. Some people take diuretics only when they feel they ate too much salt on a particular day. This tactic can cause fluid levels to be too low, actually increasing Meniere's symptoms and potentially causing constipation. Being both constipated and dizzy is likely terrible combination. Keeping your fluid level as constant as possible with a low sodium diet goes a long way in helping to relieve the nausea and dizziness of Meniere's disease. Taking diuretics causes additional issues that you have to compensate for. For one, you need to drink plenty of fluids (64 oz. or more of water per day) because you can become dehydrated if you don't. All that water passing through your body also removes potassium which has to be replaced; usually by eating a banana or two a day, by drinking orange juice or eating a regular or sweet potato. Bananas and orange juice are not permitted on my diet (discussed in chapter 14). Diuretics also tend to put more strain on your kidneys than nature intended, so it's probably not a good idea to use them as a permanent part of your routine unless your doctor is OK with it.

Decongestant:

I also found Sudafed® (a non-drowsy decongestant) able to help alleviate some of my dizziness. I'm pretty sure that the reason I got some relief was because it helped clear my sinuses and eliminate some of the pressure changes to my inner ear. Unfortunately, Sudafed® may cause rapid heartbeat (Tachycardia) in some people, especially if it's used long term. In people who are sensitive, their heat beat may beat so fast that their heart no longer pumps blood efficiently and they pass out; requiring a trip to the emergency room.

SERC® (Betahistine Hydrochloride):

SERC® is synthetic histamine taken in pill form. SERC® is of great interest because it has provided relief for many Meniere's sufferers. What is strange about SERC® is that while my approach to eliminating my Meniere's symptoms has been to significantly reduce my histamine level, SERC® apparently provides relief by actually increasing a person's histamine level. According to Solvay Pharmaceuticals (purchased by Abbott Labs), SERC® relives dizziness by normalizing the flow of (nerve) impulses and increasing blood flow within the inner ear. They also state that SERC® was developed in Europe in the 1970's specifically for the treatment of Meniere's disease after scientists discovered that Meniere's symptoms in certain patients were reduced after receiving injections of histamine. Bee stings were actually used to create histamine in patients' before that. Since the injected histamine had unpleasant side effects (and bee stings were also very unpleasant), they developed SERC®, a synthetic form of histamine that could be taken in pill form and didn't have these side effects. One problem with SERC® is that it can cause severe hypersensitivity and allergic reactions. This is likely why it's not FDA approved and is not currently available in the United States. If you want to try it, you need to contact your European, Canadian or Mexican doctor for a prescription.

Diamine Oxidase (DAO) – Histame™/ DAOSin®:

According to Histame™ and DAOSin® advertisements; just like some people are lactose intolerant and can take Lactaid® or similar products which contain lactase enzymes to help them digest milk products; there are other people who are histamine intolerant. Histamine is contained in many foods and needs to be converted to another chemical in the small intestine by the DAO enzyme. If a person is DAO deficient and the histamine goes undigested, (according to the manufacturers) it can cause many problems including: runny nose, headache, digestive problems, diarrhea, heart palpitations, etc. Taking one or two pills within fifteen minutes of eating histamine rich food, are purported to resolve these problems. In reality, these products are more likely to help with stomach acidity issues than the other problems described, but to be fair they may also help those issues for some people. It's not clear if these supplements will help Meniere's symptoms. They are likely worth a try if your doctor agrees.

Chapter 10: Surgical Treatments

Minor Surgical Treatments

I call these first two solutions minor surgical treatments because they are minimally invasive. Both treatments involve placing a small hole in the ear drum. I don't know if they were available when I developed Meniere's or if they were just unknown to my doctors. I would have likely tried the Meniett® Device, since there very little risk and no permanent damage if it doesn't work (providing the hole made in the eardrum heals which they don't always). The MicroWick™ treatment on the other hand is irreversible.

Meniett® Device:

The Meniett® Device has been around for some time and was manufactured by Medtronic but now seems to be made by LiNA Medical (which may be a subsidiary). According to the meniett.com website, the device provides relief for 70% of Meniere's suffers and suggests that Meniere's disease is caused by too much endolymphatic fluid in the semi-circular canals and cochlea. The Meniett® device is used for five minutes three times a day to deliver low pressure air pulses to the ear through a small hole made in the ear drum (typically by a laser) into which a tiny vent tube is installed. This pressure somehow temporarily displaces the excess endolymph fluid reducing pressure in the inner ear and reducing Meniere's symptoms. The patient needs to wear ear plugs when swimming or when in the shower so as not to get bacteria in the hole, as well as have it checked regularly by a doctor. A six week trial period for the device was available a few years ago, but it's unclear now how the unit is purchased or if any refund is available if it doesn't work for you. The device holds promise for reducing Meniere's symptoms, but will not resolve the issue(s) causing the disease. Sources report that the unit costs about $3,500 and is rarely covered by insurance. You can occasionally find a used unit on Ebay, but it's likely not a viable purchase as the procedure to install the vent in the ear likely requires the purchase of a new machine from the doctor performing the procedure. I would also consider the use of a used machine very risky due to the risk of bacterial contamination entering the ear.

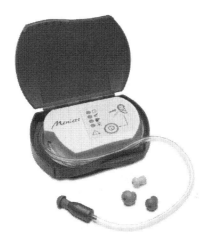

Meniett® Device
(Image Courtesy of and Copyright © Medtronic, Inc.
Meniett® is a Registered Trademark of Medtronic Inc.)

MicroWick™:

The Silverstein MicroWick™ treatment (named after its inventor Dr. Herbert Silverstein) is essentially a substantial improvement on the Transtympanic Gentamicin Injection treatment (discussed below). According to their web site, it has high success rate in eliminating dizziness and a better than average success rate in reducing ear pressure and tinnitus. Although, apparently a small percentage of people who have the treatment loose some or all of their hearing in the treated ear, it is still much better than the 20% chance of hearing loss for the Transtympanic Gentamicin Injection procedure which is described later.

The treatment is performed by making a hole in the ear drum with a CO_2 laser. A tiny plastic tube is inserted in the hole. A wick is then inserted in the tube until it rests on the duct to the inner ear. The patient drips dilute Gentamicin (a powerful antibiotic) solution in their ear three times a day for two to three weeks. The solution travels through the wick directly into the inner ear. The Gentamicin destroys the tiny hair like fibers in the problem ear that are transmitting the faulty balance signals to the brain. This allows the balance organ in the "good" ear to take over, eventually reducing or eliminating dizziness. Unfortunately, if the balance problem later develops in the other "good" ear, it's a problem.

I sent an email to Dr. Silverstein's office (many years ago) with a few questions that I would like answered if I were going to have the procedure. The questions and answers I received from Seth Rosenberg MD FACS, Ear Research Foundation Sarasota, Florida are shown below:

Q: Does the medication delivered by MicroWick™ eventually destroy the balance center in the ear like a direct Gentamicin injection? A: Yes.

Q: When you medicate yourself, do you feel dizzy for a time? A: You may feel imbalance temporarily.

Q: Is it painful? A: No!

Q: Does the device eventually get removed? A: Yes.

Q: Does the hole always repair itself? A: Usually.

Q: How do you shower with the device in your ear? A: The ear is blocked with cotton.

Q: Can't any liquid that enters cause serious infection? A: Rarely.

Q: Does the wick get dirty and need to be replaced? A: No.

Q: How often does the wick fall out or in? A: Rarely.

Major Surgical Treatments

The specialists I went to for treatment offered me three barbaric surgical options. Despite my suffering I considered them completely unacceptable for me, although in all fairness they have helped many others. The existence of these treatments provides proof that medical science is still in its infancy.

The Spinal Shunt:

It is believed that Meniere's disease is caused by an excess of endolymph fluid in the (problem) inner ear. If the fluid level can't be controlled in any other way, your doctor might suggest the spinal shunt operation which has been available for many years. Essentially the spinal shunt is an elaborate and delicate surgery that places an overflow valve in your "defective" inner ear. When the level of balance fluid in your inner ear becomes too high, the excess flows through a tiny surgically implanted pipe added to your spinal column where the fluid drains into the existing spinal fluid. I don't have statistics available, but apparently this treatment has only a moderate success rate of relieving Meniere's symptoms. However, it has provided relief for many people. This surgery requires opening of the skull which makes it an extremely serious operation, probably requiring a day or so in intensive care and a few days in the hospital after the surgery. The surgery may have to be repeated if the other inner ear becomes problematic.

Transtympanic Gentamicin Injection (TTG):

Both the TTG and Vestibular Neurectomy techniques are very similar in terms of their objective which is to prevent faulty balance nerve impulses from your damaged inner ear from getting to your brain.

In the Transtympanic Gentamicin Injection procedure (which is done in the doctor's office), the defective inner ear is injected with Gentamicin through the ear drum into the inner ear. Gentamicin destroys the tiny hairs that transmit balance information to the brain, essentially instantly destroying the "defective" balance organ. This techniques causes days (or even weeks) of profound dizziness, but eventually the brain and body compensate for the loss by relying on the other vestibular organ. Vestibular therapy (more on that later) may be required in order to help the patient's other vestibular organ adjust more quickly and reduce dizziness symptoms caused by the procedure. The injection procedure may need to be done several times to kill all the tiny hair cells. In 80 to 85% of the cases, dizziness is eventually eliminated. Unfortunately there is a 20% chance of total hearing loss in the injected ear each time the procedure is done. MicroWick™ (discussed previously) would seem to be a better alternative to accomplish the same result.

Vestibular Nerve Section (Vestibular Neurectomy):

Vestibular Nerve Section is a surgical procedure in which the vestibular nerve that transmits signals from the balance center of the inner ear to the brain is cut where it connects to the brainstem. This operation was first performed in 1904. This technique causes days (or even weeks) of profound dizziness, but eventually the brain and body compensate for the loss by relying on the other vestibular organ. Vestibular therapy may be required in order to help the patient's other vestibular organ adjust more quickly. Apparently this procedure "cures" 95% of the people who have it done. This is a serious operation where the skull needs to be opened, so a day or so in intensive care and a few days in the hospital after the surgery are required. Risks for this procedure include possible hearing loss, facial muscle weakness and brainstem injury. Also it's possible for some of the nerves to remain uncut or even grow back causing the dizziness to remain or return. In one form of this procedure (the Retrosigmoid approach), 25% of patients reported severe headaches that required medication as long as two years after the surgery. The Transtympanic Gentamicin Injection procedure (above) is replacing this operation due to its much lower risk. MicroWick™ would seem to be an even better alternative.

There is a major problem with Transtympanic Gentamicin Injection, Vestibular Nerve Section (and even the Microwick™ treatment) that wasn't originally mentioned by my doctor. What had caused the balance problem in my right ear was unknown. If I had any of these procedures done, what would happen to me if I had a future problem with the vestibular organ in my other ear? The answer was that it was possible that my symptoms might reoccur or even worse that I would have little balance at all and be left permanently "floating". However, to be fair, these procedures have been of benefit to many people.

Chapter 11: Vestibular Therapy

In some cases a doctor or balance specialist will recommend that you engage in vestibular therapy in order to help you recover from a balance disorder. Vestibular therapy works by having you perform motions that are intended to make you dizzy while at the same time making you focus on your body position and coordination. This helps to train your brain and body to compensate for lost balance more quickly than if you were just performing normal day to day activities[4]. The therapy "exercises" can be performed at home or at a vestibular therapy center. Exercises at the center are usually more elaborate than can be done at home (such as standing on, then as you progress, slightly bouncing on a trampoline) and are theoretically more effective. It is advisable not to take any medication for dizziness during the performance of the vestibular therapy exercises. In fact, it's best not to take dizziness medications at all, or if you do need them, take them as little as possible. This is because these medications inhibit your brain and body's ability to train itself to compensate for your balance problem, prolonging your long term suffering.

The brain is remarkable for its ability to compensate for balance loss and can compensate for any (one time) loss no matter how severe (even without therapy) within a few weeks to a few months. Vestibular therapy

---

[4] I use the words "brain and body" here instead of just brain because balance isn't only controlled by the brain. There are two Vestibulospinal Tracts that connect from each balance organ to the spinal cord and down through the entire body. These tracts are responsible for the instantaneous control of various muscles in the body that keep us balanced.

and not taking dizziness medications accelerates the compensation process.

Vestibular therapy is not just limited to balance exercises. Some therapy centers can diagnose which ear is causing your balance issue and even perform the Epley Maneuver which has a very good chance of curing individuals suffering from Benign Paroxysmal Positional Vertigo (BPPV) also called Benign Positional Vertigo (BPV), discussed later.

You also compensate for balance loss in other ways. Your brain may rely much more on your vision and muscle feedback to determine your position and how you are moving through space. Early into my Meniere's recovery I noticed that I became dizzy and off balance in a dark room. In fact, I could hardly walk without tipping over and needed to support myself by holding onto furniture and touching the wall. When the lights were turned on, miraculously I had much of my balance back. Amazingly, my brain used my vision to compensate for my balance loss.

Vestibular Exercises:

One of the doctors I saw specializing in balance disorders gave me these exercises to perform. I believe they were developed in the 1940's. They should be performed several times a day while not medicated if possible. Exercises should be done according to your ability, while always pushing yourself a little. If some exercises make you too dizzy, work up to them. You should do them more slowly or with less repetitions, etc. Have someone help you if necessary to avoid injury.

Cawthorne's Vestibular Exercises:

Eye Exercises	Looking up, then down. Slowly at first then quickly (20 times). Looking side to side. Slowly at first then quickly (20 times). Focus on a finger while at arm's length. Move the finger one foot closer and back again (20 times).
Head Exercises	Bend your head slowly forward then backward slowly with eyes open, then more quickly (20 times). Turn head from side to side slowly with eyes open, then more quickly (20 times). As dizziness decreases, do this exercise with your eyes closed.
Sitting	While sitting, shrug shoulders (20 times). Turn shoulders right then left (20 times). Bend forward and pick up objects from the ground and sit up (20 times).
Standing	Change from sitting to standing and back again with eyes open (20 times). Repeat with eyes closed. Throw a small rubber ball from hand to hand above eye level. Throw ball from hand to hand under one knee.

Moving About	Walk across the room with eyes open, then closed (10 times). Walk up and down a slope with eyes open, then closed (10 times). Walk up and down steps with eyes open, then closed (10 times). Observe caution and have someone help you so you don't injure yourself!
	Any game involving stooping or turning is good.

Brandt-Daroff Vestibular Exercises:

This exercise is probably not possible for many people with BPPV although that's who the exercise is meant to help. The US National Institute of Health web site: https://www.ncbi.nlm.nih.gov/pubmed/22935812 indicates that this exercise is only about 43% effective in reducing symptoms when done for several weeks vs. 93% for the Epley maneuver which is typically done for just one session. Despite the relative ineffectiveness of this exercise I present it here for both completeness and the fact that your ENT will likely give you a poorly photo copied sheet with this exercise on it.

The exercise is performed as follows:

Repeat these steps five times per session. Sessions should be 3 times per day for two weeks.

- Sit on the side of a bed in the center with your legs on the floor.

- Lie down on one side and turn your head so you are looking at the ceiling. Stay like this for 30 seconds.

- Return to the initial sitting position and stay in that position for 30 seconds.

- Lie down on your other side as before for 30 seconds.

- Return to the initial sitting position and stay in that position for 30 seconds.

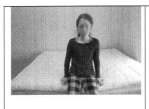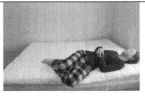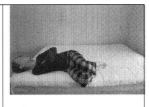

The Three Brandt-Daroff Positions

Chapter 12: Histamine Problem

Neither the doctors nor the balance specialists could provide me with a cure for my balance disorder or even an explanation as to why I had it. Finally, I went to see a biochemist nutritionist, who by using a sophisticated blood test (then called a Blood Plasma Analysis or Depression Platelet Profile) quickly discovered my problem. I had an unbelievably high histamine level, the fifth highest he had ever seen. He told me that high histamine was very likely the cause of my balance problem and Meniere's symptoms. This histamine-balance connection seems to have been confirmed by over ten years of emails send by suffers to my Balance Disorder web site. Many people diagnosed with Meniere's disease or a balance disorder in general, probably have a high histamine level causing or aggravating their dizziness symptoms. If true, like me, these people should be able to obtain substantial relief from their dizziness symptoms by reducing their body's abnormally high histamine level. How this is done is explained in this book.

Based on my nutritionist's analysis of my blood work, he was actually able to guess the symptoms I was having. These symptoms are typical of a person with a very high histamine level. He was so accurate, it was as amazing. My symptoms included: itchy skin especially on my back, lots of nervous energy (vibrating my legs while sitting) followed by periods of tiredness or exhaustion, panic attacks, difficulty focusing and with memory.

What is Histamine?

Histamine is a chemical in the blood stream that acts as a neurotransmitter and is involved in immune response. The quantity of histamine in the blood stream increases due to an allergic reaction caused by various allergens a person is exposed to. Allergens may include: pollen, dog dander, mosquito bites, various foods, etc. When you get a mosquito bite, your body reacts by releasing additional histamine which collects in the area of the bite increasing blood flow to that area, making your skin red, itchy and causing it to swell. Histamine helps your body fight cellular damage, foreign cells and proteins or particles that have entered your body. In extreme cases, the histamine level in someone who is allergic to bee venom or a particular food like strawberries for example, can become so high that anaphylactic shock and possibly death can result within minutes. Epinephrine (Adrenaline) is the only chemical that can immediately eliminate histamine in the human body. If someone is in danger of going into anaphylactic shock (where their organs shut down), it is essential that they be injected with Epinephrine (typically with an EpiPen®) immediately to counteract the dangerously high histamine level and prevent death. Sometimes people have a severe allergic reaction to an allergy shot. After the allergy shot is given, the allergist will always make the patient sit in the waiting room for about ten minutes. This is because, if the patient does have a severe reaction, Epinephrine can be injected immediately to counteract it. You might think the person could just take an antihistamine in the event of an allergic reaction. Unfortunately the answer is yes and no. Antihistamines like Benadryl® only work to block some of the body's histamine receptors, relieving or subduing some symptoms; so taking Benadryl®

53

will help to a point. Unfortunately, antihistamines do not actually remove any histamine from the body like Epinephrine and so they are helpful, but not sufficient for potentially life threatening allergic reactions or for fully eliminating histamine induced Meniere's symptoms.

Histamine is not just created by the body, but is also contained in many foods. The histamine contained in foods is "digested" in the small intestine by an enzyme called Diamine Oxidase (DAO). If not enough of the histamine is broken down by the DAO, it can cause excess stomach acid and Gastric Reflux. Gastric Reflux is acid that escapes from the stomach into the throat (esophagus) causing "Heart Burn". The "undigested" histamine can also enter the blood stream, adding to the histamine your body produces on its own. This is why Histame™ and DAOSin® discussed previously may help some Meniere's sufferers.

Histamine and Adrenaline:

My blood test indicated that my histamine level was much higher than normal but not dangerously (anaphylactic shock) high. However, the level was apparently high enough to be the cause of my Meniere's and panic attack symptoms.

Normally the body produces a certain amount of adrenaline. The amount produced increases or decreases to balance your body's changing histamine level. My body tried to reduce my extremely high histamine, by releasing larger than normal amounts of adrenaline into my blood stream. This extra adrenaline had the effect of giving me lots of nervous energy. I had trouble sitting still and my leg(s) would vibrate in an attempt to burn off the extra energy. Occasionally, my body would release abnormally large bursts of adrenalin, which caused me to have panic attacks. Two or three times a day, in its futile attempt to reduce my histamine level to normal, my body would temporarily use up its supply of adrenaline. This would leave me feeling anywhere from a little tired to completely exhausted and drained of energy. I sometimes had the feeling that that my heart would just stop beating and I would die from exhaustion. My high histamine levels also caused difficulty thinking, focusing and remembering.

High histamine levels can sometimes be reduced if the cause of the "allergic" (or autoimmune) reaction can be found (such as an allergy to cats). Unfortunately, in my case it was determined that my high histamine was not caused by an allergic reaction, but most likely by a genetic variation causing a problem with my body's ability to metabolize histidine as well as sulfur, which is contained in almost all foods in various amounts. A small percentage of the population (including many Meniere's sufferers) also have this problem.

Histidine:

I also had an excess of an amino acid called histidine which is contained in wheat, all food containing wheat, and many other food products. Histidine converts into histamine through a process in the body that causes it to lose a single carbon dioxide molecule. Many foods contain histidine including: breads, cakes, pasta, etc. The American diet can make it very easy to "load up" on histidine. The body normally converts some of the body's histidine into histamine. In my case, histidine to histamine conversion seems to occur in my body at an abnormally high rate. The more histidine I ate, the more histamine I produced and the worse my balance problem became.

Sulfur - Why Sulfur is a Problem for Some People

Sulfur is present in almost all foods in two possible forms; as part of an amino acid and/or as the mineral itself. Sulfur containing (bound) amino acids include: Methionine, Cysteine, Homocysteine, and Taurine. Methionine is present in almost every food and is abundant in the human body. Methionine creates SAMe (S-Adenosyl Methionine) which is necessary for cells to function and causes the breakdown of Dopamine, noradrenaline, adrenaline and to a small extent, histamine as well. For simplicity, I'll just say that noradrenaline and adrenaline affect the body's energy level. Dopamine is a neurotransmitter which affects memory, learning, mood, personality and many other things. In sensitive people (like myself), too much sulfur produces too much SAMe which breaks down too much Dopamine adversely affecting memory and mood. It also breaks down noradrenaline and adrenaline too rapidly making the levels of these chemicals abnormally low decreasing my energy level. A low adrenaline level allows histamine to increase, affecting the body's histamine/ adrenaline balance. Excess histamine can cause many problems which can include causing or exacerbating Meniere's disease symptoms.

To reduce my sulfur and histamine level, I had to eliminate foods from my diet that contained high sulfur content as well as those (like wheat) that contained high amounts of histidine. If I ate a few slices of pizza which has tomato sauce (which contains sulfur), crust (wheat which contains histidine), and cheese (which contains histidine) I would usually become dizzy in two or three days because it took that long for the sulfur, histidine, histamine reaction to take place. I would never have associated a dizziness attack with something I ate two or three days before, nor would most people.

I believe that the key to significantly reducing the symptoms of Meniere's disease is to avoid foods that contain histidine, histamine and high sulfur content as much as possible. The following is a list of foods high in sulfur that as a Meniere's suffer I try to avoid:

High Methionine (Sulfur) Containing Foods

All fish	Bean sprouts	Beer	Brazilnuts
Cabbage	Celery	Coleslaw	Collard Greens
Cranberries	Dandelion greens	Dried Fruits (with Sulfur based preservatives, i.e. Sulfites)	Endive
Garlic	Ginger	Grapes	Green, Red, Yellow Peppers
Grapefruit	Hard Liquors	Kale	Kelp Seaweed
Lemon	Leeks	Lime	Miso soup
Okra	Onions	Oranges	Peanuts
Peanut butter	Peas	Poppy seeds	Pumpkin seeds
Raisins	Rice (White or Brown)	Sesame seeds	Soy beans
Soy sauce	Sunflower seeds	Swiss chard	Tahini
Tangerines	Tamari Sauce	Tofu	Tofutti
Turnips	Wakame Seaweed	Wines	

I also avoid all food and beverages with preservatives that contain sulfur, sulfur dioxide, potassium metabisulfite, sulfites and sulfates.

Note that although fish (for example), probably should be avoided due to its high sulfur content, its dietary benefits far outweigh its problems and so it is included as a small part of my diet. This link is a good resource for food Sulfur content:

http://apjcn.nhri.org.tw/server/info/books-phds/books/foodfacts/html/data/data5g.html

The following is a list of food high in histamine and/ or histidine that I try to avoid:

Histamine and Histidine Containing Foods

All Dairy Products	Crackers from Wheat	Pasta	Soups with Tomato base
All Milk and Milk Products	Cream	Pigeon Peas	Soups from Milk
Bananas	Cream Sauces	Pineapple	Sour Cream
Black Beans	Edam	Pinto Beans	Spaghetti Sauces
Blue Cheese	Eggplant	Powdered Milk	Spinach
Bread (with Wheat)	French Dressing	Protein drinks with Whey or Casein	Strawberries
Cakes made with wheat	Granola Bars	Red Wines	Taco Chips
Cheeses	Havarti	Ricotta	Tomato
Chicken Livers	Oatmeal	Russian Dressing	Wheat Products
Corn Chips	Oats	Salami (Genoa)	

Chapter 13: Blood Plasma Analysis

The blood plasma test that discovered my histamine problem was done by a (now defunct) lab that specialized in histamine testing and was called a "Depression Platelet Profile". The test was ordered by my nutritionist. The blood was drawn at my primary care physician's office. They obtained the special test tubes and detailed instructions for the test in advance from the test lab. The test required a 24 hour fast (not eating) and avoiding all chemicals including: soap, toothpaste, and deodorant. Use of any of these products could affect the test results. The blood test profiled my neurotransmitter and various amino-acids levels.

Where to get the blood test done (now):

Proving you can find a biochemist/ nutritionist who can interpret the results, the only lab I know of that can perform this unique blood test (called the Amino Acid Profile and Amine Scan) is:

Health Diagnostics and Research Institute (H.D.R.I) - formally Vitamin Diagnostics

540 Bordentown Avenue, Suite 2300 South Amboy, NJ 08879

Tel: +1 732-721-1234; Fax: +1 732-525-3288

Chapter 14: Meniere's Diet

Low Sodium

A low salt diet of 1,000-1,200 mg of sodium or less per day is the generally accepted dietary method for controlling Meniere's disease. Keeping a consistently low sodium level can be very effective in helping to alleviate dizziness. Salt intake during the day should be spaced out as evenly as possible. Ingesting very little salt during most of the day then having 800 mg of sodium in a microwave dinner will probably make you dizzy. It is also helps to keep your water intake spaced out evenly throughout the day, drinking 64 oz. (8 - 8 oz. glasses) or more per day. Water consumption should be increased if using a diuretic and to keep pace with sweating caused by hot weather or exercise. If you want to go to extremes, experiment and keep records to find out how much water is makes you feel your best. Record how dizzy you feel each day and drink the amount of water that works best for you.

A low salt (sodium) diet essentially means giving up or limiting your intake of several food "varieties" including those below. You very quickly get used to eating low sodium foods. After a short time you will find "normally" salted food to be almost inedible.

- Frozen microwave dinners and prepared foods: Even so called healthy, diet or low calorie dinners contain frighteningly high quantities of sodium, many as high as 800 mg. Almost no frozen dinners or bagged foods are acceptable on a Meniere's diet. Check the labels. Be in for a shock.

- Soups: Most canned soups have incredibly high levels of sodium. I'm almost surprised that the cans don't rust from the inside out. Fortunately low sodium soups have recently become available.

- Snack Foods (chips, popcorn, salted nuts and alike): They contain very large amounts of salt and should be avoided.

- Cheese: Most cheese contains enormous amounts of salt. In cheese making, the cheese is dumped into salt vats to stop (kill) the bacteria used in its production. (Alpine Lace low salt cheese might be fine in small amounts).

- Chinese, Japanese, Mexican and other regional foods: These foods are commonly prepared with large amounts of salt. Although you can ask the restaurant to not add any salt, they will still cook with traditional sauces such as Soy sauce which are rich in sodium. Steamed is about the best you can do at a Chinese restaurant, although some restaurants do have a low sodium menu. Also avoid MSG!

- Fast Foods: These are typically very high in sodium although there are a few exceptions. Fast food restaurants are required to post their food's nutritional information on a poster in the restaurant so be sure to look for it. It's usually posted on a mostly hidden wall somewhere in the dining area as it's designed to blend into the scenery. You can order French fries with no salt at some restaurants. Unfortunately they are almost always made with lots of salt anyway. They just don't sprinkle extra on top.

- French Fries: Nearly all brands of frozen French Fries, especially those used in restaurants are made with high quantities of salt (baked in). Amounts of 250 - 425 mg per serving are common. Some generic or supermarket brands only contain 25 mg or so per serving, so if you like fries, look for these. Avoid all others.
- Added Salt: Avoid adding salt to foods like French Fries, soup, pop-corn, etc.
- Condiments and Sauces: Soy and Teriyaki sauce, salad dressings and many other condiments contain surprising amounts of sodium. Check the labels.

The US Department of Agriculture (USDA) publishes a database that contains a comprehensive listing of the ingredients and chemical composition of an enormous number of foods, including fast foods, breakfast foods, etc. It will help you determine how much salt is in the foods you eat. It also details sugar and other chemicals. Check their web site for the database. http://ndb.nal.usda.gov/

The Low Histamine, Low Histidine, Reduced Sulfur, Low Sodium, No Sugar Diet

My diet is designed to reduce my intake of histamine, histidine, sulfur, sodium and eliminate sugar (sucrose). As previously discussed, the purpose in reducing histamine, histidine and sulfur is to decrease and balance the body's histamine level. Reducing sodium is a widely accepted and necessary step in controlling the symptoms of any balance disorder. This diet is the reason I rarely suffer from Meniere's symptoms. It can help you too (if your doctor agrees).

It was important (at least initially) when I started my low histamine diet to completely eliminate sugar. This is because sugar causes the body to release adrenaline shortly after ingesting it. Many parents have noticed that their children become "very energetic" after eating sugar. This is because sugar gives them an adrenaline boost. If your histamine level is high, two things may happen when you eat sugar. The first is that your adrenaline level may spike causing lots of nervous energy, worsening dizziness symptoms, and possibly even causing a panic attack. The second is that the sugar, by causing your body to release more adrenaline than is needed, may exhaust its already low supply. This causes periods of very low energy or even exhaustion. Fruit sugar (fructose), honey, NutraSweet®, Saccharin, and <u>real</u> maple syrup won't increase your adrenaline level, so they can be used instead of sugar.

My Diet

The initial diet I was on for many months to control my balance problem is presented below. This diet was created specifically <u>for me</u> by my nutritionist using the data obtained from my blood tests. It can be used as a model to control your Meniere's or balance disorder symptoms, <u>but it is essential that you discuss it with your doctor and have all appropriate testing done, before you consider emulating it.</u>

<u>A diet that was helpful for me may be harmful for you!</u>

My diet is very high in protein and contains a substantial amount of meat and eggs, which are alleged to cause high cholesterol. I have discovered (at least for me), that this is apparently not true. Despite being on this diet or minor variations of it for years, my cholesterol level was 120 to 133 which is low normal. The key is to eat high quality, low fat cuts of meat and avoid hamburgers. Also eating a handful of cashew nuts and a handful of walnuts every day reduces cholesterol levels as does the niacin I took (see the chapter on supplements). As it turns out, high cholesterol is apparently caused by baked goods like cakes, cookies and breads which I try my best to avoid.

Sugar is addictive, so I did feel the "withdrawal" for a few days after I stopped eating it. Early into the diet I accidently ate some sugar that was in a salad dressing. I became extremely jittery and was a bit concerned until I realized what had happened. Now that my histamine level is significantly reduced, sugar doesn't affect me.

Getting the diet started was a serious business for me. I was suffering so much that changing my diet became the top priority in my life. I completely cleaned out my kitchen cabinets of everything I was not supposed to eat. I threw out all my microwave dinners. I went to a meat store and purchased a week's worth of meat, as the diet is broken down that way. I stocked up on everything else at the supermarket.

My most recent diet is also shown below. It is very similar to the one I was on over twenty years ago.

My Initial Diet:

Meats 5 to 8 oz. Portions: Lunch & Dinner

Meat	Times/ week	Notes:
Beef	2	As lean as possible (avoid burgers)
Pork	4	As lean as possible (no bacon or sausage)
Chicken	3	No breading allowed (avoid fried)
Turkey	4	Contains: Tryptophan
Fish	1	Anything from the sea is ok.

Fruit: 5 Times per Day

Apples	Apricots	Blueberries	Blackberries	Cantaloupe
Coconut	Dates	Figs	Honeydew	Kiwi
Mangos	Nectarines	Papaya	Peaches	Pears
Plums	Prunes	Raspberries	Watermelon	Jennies Macaroons

Vegetables: Two 8 oz. Cups per Day

Alfalfa Sprouts	Artichoke	Asparagus	Avocado
Beets	Broccoli	Carrots	Cauliflower
Chickpeas	Cucumber	Kidney Beans	Lettuce (Boston)
Lettuce (Chicory)	Lettuce (Iceberg)	Lettuce (Romaine)	Lentils
Leeks	Lima Beans	Mushrooms	Onions
Potatoes	Radishes	Scallions	Sweet Potato
String Beans	Squash	Zucchini	

Grains (2 Slices of bread only allowed per day)

Rye Bread
Pumpernickel

Eggs: Two per Day

Nuts & Seeds (Essential for Good Cholesterol Balance)
One Cup of each per Week

Cashews	Non-Salted, Raw or Roasted.
Walnuts	Non-Salted.

Condiments:

Newman's Own Dressing	Sesame Oil	Mayonnaise (Regular)	Mustard
Corn Oil	Fructose	Pepper	Olive Oil
Honey	Oil & Vinegar	Margarine	Canola Oil
All Spices (No Salt)			

Beverages:

Beverage	Quantity	Notes:
Water	(8) 8 oz. Glasses per Day	Minimum
Decaff Coffee/ Tea	As Desired	Splash of milk only allowed.
Fruit Juices	As Desired	From list of fruits above only. Juice does not count as a fruit serving.
Seltzers	As Desired	Non-Salted. Fructose base only
Soda	Up to 2 Cans per Day	NutraSweet® or Fructose only

Notes:

No milk products allowed except for a splash in coffee, etc.
No sugar allowed until histamine level is sufficiently low.
No wheat products allowed.
No tomato based products allowed.
No red or green peppers.
Avoid anything preserved with Sulfur Dioxide or equivalent.
Eat only what is on the diet, no exceptions.
Don't drink anything with caffeine.
Avoid MSG.
Spices while allowed may aggravate Meniere's symptoms. If they do avoid them.
Meat protein is only metabolized when carbohydrates are also eaten. If you ate a pound of lean meat per day and no carbohydrates, you would likely starve. The limited carbohydrates in this diet allow for the large consumption of meat.

My Recent Maintenance Diet:

Meats 5 to 8 oz. Portions: Lunch & Dinner

Meat	Times/ week	Notes:
Beef	2	As lean as possible (avoid burgers)
Pork	3	As lean as possible (no bacon or sausage)
Chicken	3	No breading allowed (avoid fried)
Turkey	4	Contains: Tryptophan
Fish	2	Anything from the sea is ok.

Fruit: 4 Times per Day

Apples	Apricots	Cantaloupe	Casaba Melon	Coconut
Crenshaw Melon	Dates	Grapefruit	Grapes	Guava
Honeydew	Mangos	Nectarines	Oranges	Papaya
Peaches	Pears	Plums	Prunes	Star fruit
Tangerines	Tangelos	Watermelon		

Vegetables: Two 8 oz. Cups per Day

Alfalfa Sprouts	Artichoke	Asparagus	Avocado
Beets	Broccoli	Carrots	Cauliflower
Cucumber	Lettuce (Boston)	Lettuce (Chicory)	Lettuce (Iceberg)
Lettuce (Romaine)	Leeks	Mushrooms	Onions
Radishes	Scallions	String Beans	Squash
Potatoes	Zucchini		

Grains (2 Slices of bread only allowed per day)

Rye Bread or Pumpernickel
Soba noodles (100% buckwheat), Two 8 oz. cups per week.

Eggs: Two Omega 3 Eggs per day

Nuts & Seeds (Essential for Good Cholesterol Balance)

One 8 oz. Cup of each per Week

Almond Butter
Cashew Butter

Condiments:

Vinaigrette Dressing	Fructose	Margarine (Smart Balance)	Mustard
Canola Oil	Corn Oil	Olive Oil	Sesame Oil
Walnut Oil	Pepper	Oil & Vinegar	Honey
All Spices* (No Salt)		Mayonnaise (Regular)	

Beverages:

Beverage	Quantity	Notes:
Water	(10) 8 oz. Glasses per Day	
Decaff Coffee/ Tea	As desired	Splash of milk only allowed.
Fruit Juices	As desired	From list of fruits above only. Juice does not count as a fruit serving.
Seltzers	As desired	Non-Salted. Fructose base only.
Soda	1 to 2 cans per day	NutraSweet® or Fructose Only

Notes:

No milk products allowed except for a splash in coffee, etc.
No sugar allowed until histamine level is sufficiently low.
No wheat products allowed.
No tomato based products allowed.
No red or green peppers.
Avoid anything preserved with Sulfur Dioxide or equivalent.
Eat only what is on the diet, no exceptions.
Don't drink anything with caffeine.
Avoid MSG.
Spices while allowed may aggravate Meniere's symptoms. If they do avoid them.

Chapter 15: Supplements

Based on my symptoms and blood work, my former nutritionist "prescribed" the following supplements. The supplements and their dosage were periodically adjusted (every six months or so) based on additional blood work, how I felt, and environmental conditions. For example, during allergy season or the winter (when the noxious fumes emitted from oxygenated gasoline are present) I may take more niacin.

While it may be tempting to just start using these supplements to help control your Meniere's symptoms, it is essential that you discuss them with your doctor and have all appropriate testing done before taking them. It is also essential that your doctor monitor you while taking them. Drug (or supplement) induced Hepatitis (leading to liver failure) is always a possibility when taking any supplement. Supplements are not regulated by the FDA (Federal Drug Administration) and have their own risks as I unfortunately discovered.

The supplement, dosage and function of each are shown in the table below:

My Initial Supplements

Supplement	Dosage/ Day	Effect
Vitamin C	1000 mg/ (3 x)	Removes toxins including: nitrates, nitrites, sulfites. Helps prevent colds. Aids the immune system.
Vitamin B Complex Includes 40 mg of B3	2 Capsules/ (3x)	Cofactor for many amino acid reactions. Helps cellular pumping action to control fluid level in cells. Supposed to help improve the nervous system function. Niacin/ Niacinamide and Nicotinic acid is also contained in B-Complex.
Beta Carotene	11,000 I.U./ (1x)	For anticancer
Multi-Minerals	2 Capsules/ (3x)	Provides mineral essentials including calcium at many times the amount of a multi-vitamin.
Niacin/ Niacinamide	200 mg / 200 mg (3x)	Niacin (B3) Removes histamine from the body.
L-Serine	500 mg/ (2 x)	Partially cuts off adrenaline surges. Allows noradrenaline and dopamine levels to increase.
Norival 300 mg	2 Capsules/ (2x)	Digestible tyrosine. Produces dopamine, noradrenaline and adrenaline.
L-Glutamine	500 mg/ (3x)	Controls balance and coordination of the body in time and space.
NADH	3.6 mg/ (2x)	Helps cellular electron transport. Reported to help increase energy, and is an antioxidant.

My After 20 years Maintenance Supplements

Supplement	Dosage/ Day	Effect
Vitamin C	1000 mg/ (3 x)	Removes toxins including: nitrates, nitrites, sulfites. Helps prevent colds. Aids the immune system.
Vitamin B Complex Includes 40 mg of B3	2 Capsules/ (3x)	Cofactor for many amino acid reactions. Helps cellular pumping action to control fluid level in cells. Supposed to help improve the nervous system function. Niacin/ Niacinamide and Nicotinic acid is also contained in B-Complex.
Beta Carotene	11,000 I.U./ (1x)	For anticancer
D3	1,000 I.U./ (1x)	Helps the immune system.
Multi-Minerals	2 Capsules/ (3x)	Provides mineral essentials including calcium at many times the amount of a multi-vitamin.
Norival 300 mg	2 Capsules/ (3x)	Digestible tyrosine. Produces dopamine, noradrenaline and adrenaline.
Quercitin 500 mg	1 Capsule/ mg (3x)	Anti-oxidant, Anti-inflammatory, Anti-histamine. Balances histamine level.
Phosphodytal Choline 840 mg	1 Capsule/ (3x)	Helps to promote healthy cognitive function.
Black Current Seed Oil 500 mg	2 Capsules (3x)	Fatty Acid to raise good cholesterol.

Note:

The supplements shown above were prescribed specifically for me based on my recent blood test results. I decided on the supplements below myself after my nutritionist "retired".

Consult your doctor before considering taking any supplements!

What I take now (and it works for me)

Supplement	Dosage/ Day	Effect
Multivitamin	1 x per day	Supposed to support overall health.
D3	1,000 I.U./ (1x) per day	Helps the immune system.
Niacin (Nicotinic acid)	125mg (1x) per day	Removes Histamine from the body.

Niacin

The best way to remove histamine from the body (aside from an epinephrine injection) is to take niacin or a B-Complex vitamin containing it. Unfortunately, after taking niacin, you may experience something called a "Niacin flush". A flush is caused by the dilation (expansion) of blood vessels which increases the amount of blood flow to the skin. A flush can occur within a few minutes of taking niacin, although it may not occur every time. A mild flush will cause the skin to turn red and become itchy. It starts at the top of the head and travels quickly down the entire length of the body.

The intensity of a flush tends to increase with the level of histamine in the body. If you have a very high histamine level, the flushes can be significantly more "painful" depending on the quantity of niacin you ingest. Histamine resides in large quantities in the skin, lungs, sinuses, stomach and intestines. The flush can cause your skin to feel very warm or even hot, like it's burning. It can also cause your lungs to feel like they are burning; cause difficulty breathing, stomach pains, vomiting, and diarrhea. A flush can be made worse by bathing or showering just before or while you are having one. A flush can last from about five to thirty minutes and while possibly painful, it's not harmful and won't cause any "long term" damage (unless your doctor tells you differently). If flushes are too severe to be tolerated, the amount of niacin or B-Complex taken should be reduced. It's reported that taking an aspirin about one half hour before taking niacin reduces the flush. Again, discuss that with your doctor.

Note: If you have an embolism, taking niacin may be dangerous.

Check with your doctor!

There is strong evidence to suggest that niacin lowers serum cholesterol, low-density lipoprotein (a.k.a. LDL or "Bad" Cholesterol), and triglycerides, and that it raises high-density lipoprotein cholesterol (a.k.a. HDL or "Good" Cholesterol) levels which is certainly a beneficial effect for many people. The pharmaceutical industry, realizing niacin's benefits, created a prescription time release version called Niaspan™.

Only niacin which is vitamin B3 (nicotinic acid) will reduce histamine levels in the body and also cause a flush. No-Flush niacin, nicotinamide also called niacinamide or nicotinic-acid-amide will not. It's important when purchasing B-Complex or niacin supplements to check the label to make sure it contains the desired quantity of B3 (nicotinic acid). Also, the labels on some supplements do not distinguish between nicotinic acid and nicotinamide. If they don't, you can call the manufacturer who is obligated by law to tell you.

There is evidence that taking high levels of Nicotinamide, which is present many times with niacin in B-Complex supplements, can cause liver damage in some individuals and cause problems if you have an embolism, so it's important to check with a doctor's before taking it.

Taking Supplements with a Cold

When I'm coming down with a cold, I don't take niacin because it (violently) removes histamine from my body usually causing a very painful "flush". The body needs histamine to help fight the cold. Instead I used to take the following subset of my usual supplements to aid with my cold recovery.

Supplement	Dosage/ Day	Effect
Vitamin C	1000 mg/ (3 x)	Removes toxins including: nitrates, nitrites, sulfites. Helps prevent colds. Aids the immune system.
Multi-Minerals	2 Capsules/ (3x)	Provides mineral essentials including calcium at many times the amount of a multi-vitamin.
Beta Carotene	11,000 I.U./ (1x)	For anticancer
D3	1,000 I.U./ (1x)	Helps the immune system.

Notes on Supplements:

While each supplement I was given was meant to help correct deficiencies in my blood chemistry and reduce my various symptoms, the most important supplement for my Meniere's Disease was niacin. My diet and taking niacin alone (or B-Complex containing it) may have provided significant relief for my balance disorder symptoms as it does for me now. If your doctor is not an expert on supplements, ask him about just taking niacin. It might be a good place to start.

If you're going to take supplements every day, it's best to use high quality ones that contain no: fillers, preservatives, corn, wheat, salt, sugar or soy derivatives and that are allergy free. Taking so called "Veggie" capsules, where the capsule is made of vegetable and not animal protein (gelatin) is also advisable. The concern is that gelatin capsules could theoretically pass on Mad-Cow disease where Veggie capsules would not.

Vitamins oxidize and lose their effectiveness fairly quickly. They can last anywhere from six to nine months. Amino Acids can last up to two years. B-Complex and NADH must be refrigerated.

It's best to take supplements one hour before or one hour after eating with plenty of water.

Chapter 16: Exercising

There are two types of exercise that are essential for a healthy life: aerobic and strength training. Aerobic exercise can be running, rock climbing, using stair stepper machines, jumping rope, tennis, etc. Aerobic exercise strengthens your entire cardiovascular system. A fit cardiovascular system lowers your cholesterol level, risk of heart attack and stroke, makes you feel energetic, and gives you a sense of well-being. Strength training is usually weight lifting, but can also be in the form of isometrics, traditional gym exercises like pushups and crunches, etc. Strength training as the name suggests strengthens your muscles, tendons and ligaments. Strong muscles help your body to maintain a healthy posture, avoid injury, burn calories and help you to accomplish everyday tasks. Both aerobic and strength training are even more important to the health of someone with Meniere's disease.

Being physically fit helps to subdue Meniere's symptoms. Exercising is a method for helping you to feel better (less dizzy and nauseous) as well as making you healthier. Unfortunately, the act of exercising with Meniere's can be a sickening experience. Strength training and aerobic exercise can each make you dizzy in their own way.

Weight lifting exercises such as the bench press, causes you to hold your breath, clench your jaw, change your respiration, etc. These things cause a change of pressure within your ears and a change in your blood chemistry (changing oxygen and carbon dioxide levels in your blood). The heavier the weights that are being lifted, the more your body adapts your breathing and jaw clenching to lifting them, and the dizzier you may become. When I exercised, I would feel my worst shortly after completing a weight lifting exercise. Unfortunately, I didn't find a way of totally eliminating the nausea associated with weight training; although I was able to reduce it enough so it was bearable. First, I lengthened each exercise and the rest period in between. If it normally took me 60 seconds to do ten repetitions for a particular exercise, I would slow the exercise way down so that it took much longer, double or even quadruple the time. I would allow myself to take several breaths or even try to breathe normally while performing each repetition (rep). I tried to focus on not holding my breath or clenching my jaw with each rep which isn't easy. Usually, people tend to clench their jaw and exhale as they apply force to lift a weight and inhale as they lower it. This is probably a good weight lifting technique that helps to maximize the amount of weight that a person can lift. However, the devastating nausea you feel after the exercise will convince you that my method while much less efficient is better suited for people with Meniere's. After each exercise or set, you should walk around a little, try to relax and breathe normally. This helps to stabilize your breathing, lower your blood pressure and makes your body focus on balancing itself. When you change your body position for a particular exercise (such as lying down for a bench press), you should stay in that position for a while before lifting the weight. This gives you time to adjust to your new orientation before the stress of lifting the weight. After finishing a particular lifting exercise you should try to stay in that position for a minute or so and then change your position slowly.

I found that aerobic exercise was best done on equipment such as a treadmill or stair stepper. Elliptical machines made me dizzy. Having rails to hold on to was very reassuring and occasionally necessary. I was afraid running outside would expose me to too much car exhaust and pollen as well as take me too far from my couch in the event of a balance attack. Walking or running outside may be a good option, but I would bring a cell phone and perhaps a friend the first few times.

The stair stepper machine made me dizzy during and immediately after using it. The treadmill had its own issues. When starting, it made be dizzy as my brain tried to get used to walking without going anywhere. When stopping, it was even more nauseating as my brain though it was still moving even though it was not; sort of like the feeling you get when you stop roller skating, but much worse. After the dizziness associated with using the machines subsided, I actually felt almost normal for a few hours after the exercise.

Chapter 17: Reducing your Risks with Disability Insurance

Disability insurance pays you a substantial percentage of your income if you become disabled, usually until age 65. A disability may take many (unfortunate) forms including loss of vision, hearing, both legs, both arms, intense back pain, and under certain circumstances a balance disorder. I would advise anyone with a balance disorder to try to get disability insurance. The only thing worse than being incapacitated by dizziness, is not being able to support yourself and your family because of it.

If you have been going from doctor to doctor for years trying to resolve your balance problem, it may be expensive, difficult, or impossible to get insurance. During the application process, the insurance company goes through your medical records looking for problems that may cost them money later. However, if your balance problem is new, unreported to a doctor or temporary, insurance may still be possible.

Although more expensive, "Own Occupation Insurance" is the best type of disability insurance to have. It will pay you if your disability prevents you from doing the job you have now. For example, if you injure your hands and can no longer program a computer, you will receive a full disability payment. If you don't have "Own Occupation" and can't program, the insurance company can (theoretically) set you up as a greeter at Wal-Mart or answering phones in a call center. Then, they will just pay you the difference between what you made in your computer programming job and what you earn answering phones.

Chapter 18: Voodoo Cures

What's a Voodoo cure? I consider a Voodoo cure to be any cure that seems unusual, and that has no solid scientific theory or evidence to explain why it might be effective. One example of this is the use of magnets to relieve pain. As far as I can tell, there is no (reputable) scientific evidence or theory to suggest that magnets can actually relieve pain. Yet, some people (and companies) claim that magnets do work. It is of course possible that magnets relieve pain simply because the people using them believe they do. This belief releases endorphins, retrains the way their brain responds to pain, etc. Their belief that magnets work actually provides pain relief for some people. It's also possible that the magnets are actually doing something that medical science does not yet understand to reduce pain in some people. To me, this is a Voodoo cure.

The Sea-Band ®

Sea-Bands® are the brand name for a wrist band made in the UK that is supposed to give its user relief from motion sickness primarily caused during travel. Sea-Bands® are small highly elastic wrist bands that look like they can't possibly fit on an adult wrist, but they do. In the center of each band is smooth plastic bump or stud (which the manufacturer calls a pressure knob). It's about the size of a very large green pea cut in half. The bands are worn on the wrist of both arms so that the plastic bump is pressed against the tendon (and veins) in the center of your wrist. They're not exactly comfortable, but are not so uncomfortable that you can't forget you're wearing them. Sea-Bands®

did nothing to ease my Meniere's symptoms, but they did provide my mother who also had a balance disorder with some relief while traveling.

Sea-Bands® are available at drug stores, for under $15 and less online. Sea-Bands® (are said to) work by using the principle of Nei Kuan acupressure to free the flow of Chi energy. The Sea-Bands® website provides a more scientific explanation of acupressure as well as results of clinical trials. See www.sea-band.com for more details.

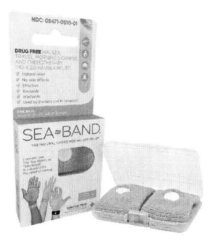

The Sea-Band®

(Image Courtesy of and Copyright Sea-Band®)

Reletex®- Formally ReliefBand®

The following text was originally written by me and modified somewhat by Neurowave, the manufacturer of the Reletex® device (in order to get permission to use their image):

"The ReliefBand®, now called Reletex® is a FDA cleared transdermal neuromodulation device for the treatment of nausea and vomiting. It uses an electronically generated pulse to stimulate the median nerve on the underside of the wrist. These signals travel to the emetic center of the brain where they act to positively modulate neural pathways, via the vagus nerve, thus restoring normal gastric rhythms. The device is supposed to help to relieve nausea caused by motion sickness. You need to apply a conductive gel to your skin so it can make good electrical contact. It has five adjustable stimulation levels. Reletex also requires a prescription which one of their distributors (http://www.aeromedixrx.com) will provide free of charge. Since I have no experience with this device, I can't say if it will work for Meniere's suffers. At this time it sells for about $95."

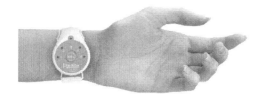

Reletex® Device

(Image Courtesy of and Copyright Neurowave Medical, Chicago, IL)

Dizziness and Tinnitus Relief Pills

There are many brands of pills on the market that claim to offer relief for Dizziness and/or Tinnitus (including a paid advertisement on the Veda.org website). Many have common Homeopathic ingredients and are taken several times a day. Some have B vitamins. One I found had a sulfur compound and another had Gingko; both of which could make matters worse. Others have Natural herbs, etc. I have no experience with these pills and have had no feedback from anyone who has tried them. Still, they may work for someone, somewhere.

SPC Flakes®

SPC Flakes® are made by POA Pharma Scandinavia AB in Sweden. According to the manufacturer, they: "stimulate the body's own production of protein AF. Antisecretory Factory (AF) is a protein that is naturally present in the body" and "can normalize fluid flow. This is of clinical significance within bowel diseases, diarrhea, Mèniére and Mastitis." Also they "must be used for approximately 14 days before the desired effect can be expected." The implied effect appears to be that these flakes may regulate endolymph in the inner ear and help with the disorder. Unfortunately I can't find any "credible" evidence this product works for Meniere's sufferers.

Miscellaneous Cures:

Over the years I have been contacted by hundreds of people in their search for a cure to their balance problem. Some have indicated they found relief through unusual methods. Others indicated methods that did not help them. I don't think that these "cures" hold much hope for Meniere's suffers, but I present them here anyway for completeness.

Upledger Institute Message

The Upledger institute teaches a very light touch message technique. It is said that this principle can help relieve a wide variety of medical problems. You can go to their website (upledger.com) to find a practitioner.

Nambudripad's Allergy Elimination Techniques

Nambudripad's Allergy Elimination Techniques (NAET®) was invented by Dr. Devi Nambudripad in 1983. It's known best for treating children with Autism. One person indicated that this technique resolved their balance disorder in about two years of treatment. According to the NAET® website, the technique desensitizes a patient to things they may be allergic to at the rate of about one allergy per treatment session, but it does not actually eliminate the allergy. For severe allergies to a particular food for example, several sessions may be required. The technique includes use of: acupressure and/ or acupuncture, kinesiologic (movement of the body), chiropractic, and nutrition. In one video on their web site, they demonstrate that part of the treatment is pressing a sealed glass vial of an allergen against the patient's arm to desensitize them to it. It would be nice to just press a bottle of aspirin against your head when you have a headache, but I have my doubts the world works like this. Still, some people may find this treatment works for them. Thousands of medical practitioners have been trained in NAET®.

Acupuncture

This ancient Chinese technique has been known to relieve a variety of ailments for many people. One Meniere's sufferer told me it helped them slightly. Others told me it was no help at all.

Acupressure

This ancient Chinese technique has also been known to relieve a variety of ailments for many people. It did not help anyone who contacted me.

Progesterone Cream

This prescription cream is used to relieve symptoms in menopausal women. One woman indicated it also helped her Meniere's symptoms. I strongly advise that you check with your doctor before trying this cream for the relief of balance disorder symptoms. Obviously, it should not be used by men!

Natrium Salicyllicum

This is a Homeopathic cure. One sufferer wrote that they felt significant relief after taking it three times per day. The medicine was administered by drinking a sip of water that has been mixed with four drops of the "medicine".

Gingko Biloba

Gingko is a well-known and well-advertised natural supplement. It is alleged to have many wonderful benefits including giving you increased energy; improving memory and making you feel less dizzy. Gingko has the effect of increasing the adrenaline level in your body for a period of time, which makes you feel temporarily more energetic. You tend to remember events that took place better when your adrenaline level is high, so Gingko can probably improve your ability to form memories. Ginkgo did absolutely nothing to help my balance disorder. In fact, it increased the severity and frequency of the panic attacks I was having at the time. I stopped using it immediately.

Garlic

Garlic is alleged to improve balance if taken regularly. I could never really decide if it worked for me over the long term. In the short term, it seemed to make me dizzier, so I don't recommend it.

Green Tea

Green tea did not help any Meniere's suffers that contacted me.

Natural Anti-Histamines

There are many natural antihistamine supplements. They include Stinging Nettle, Brigham Tea and many others. Like regular antihistamines they may help reduce balance disorder symptoms, but are unlikely to provide significant relief.

Methylsulfonylmethane (MSM)

MSM is said to relieve allergies, constipation, diverticulosis, premenstrual syndrome (PMS), and improve mood, poor circulation, high blood pressure, reduce obesity, high cholesterol and snoring as well as have many other beneficial effects. The effect of MSM on Meniere's suffers is unknown.

Marijuana

Only one Meniere's sufferer admitted taking Marijuana for their symptoms. It did not provide them with any relief.

Cocaine

Only one Meniere's sufferer admitted taking Cocaine for their symptoms. It did not provide them with any relief.

Chapter 19: Treating Yourself Step by Step

After you've had yet another balance attack and begin to realize life as you knew it is over, you'll wonder what to do next. Having gone through it all, I suggest taking the following steps:

Make Sure it's Not Serious

Make sure your dizziness is not caused by something serious like a brain tumor, blood clot, high or low blood pressure, etc. If you're older, you especially need to rule out a serious circulatory problem of the brain. The first doctor to see (after the emergency room doctor, if you had the bad luck to end up there) is a family or primary care doctor who knows your medical history. They are probably the best to help determine if you are at immediate risk from a serious medical problem where dizziness is just a symptom.

The second doctor to see should be an Ear Nose and Throat (ENT) doctor, preferably one that specializes in balance disorders. They will be able to run tests to determine if your balance problem is an inner ear problem and not something more serious.

In some cases dizziness can be caused by hyperventilation (breathing too frequently or deeply) which unless accompanied by a panic attack may go unnoticed. While many doctors consider this a psychological condition, it (in my opinion) is most likely caused by excess histamine for which the diet and supplements in chapters 14 and 15 should be considered.

See a Balance Specialist

See a doctor who specializes in balance disorders (usually an ENT or Neurologist) to again rule out any serious condition and determine if you have Benign paroxysmal Positional Vertigo (BPPV) or Meniere's disease. BPPV can be "cured" many times by undergoing the Canalith Repositioning Maneuver such as the Epley Maneuver. In some instances these maneuvers can be done at home. However they can cause such profound dizziness that help may be needed to perform them. Instructions for the Epley Maneuver are provided in chapter 21.

Determine if Your Dizziness is Recurring

Your ENT may determine that your balance problem was likely caused by a virus. In this case you would be diagnosed with Vestibular Neuronitis or Labyrinthitis. Typically when you get this mystery inner ear virus, it's a onetime occurrence. Damage to you inner ear is done just once. If this is the case, you will slowly recover your balance as your brain learns to compensate for the damage. Vestibular therapy may help to speed the recovery process. It may take several weeks to several months for all your dizziness symptoms to subside depending on how much damage was done and how quickly your brain and body learn to compensate for the damage. If you are one of the unlucky ones that have recurring dizziness that lasts for months or years and have not been diagnosed with BPPV, you have lots of home work to do to try and find the cause.

Look for Cause of Recurring Dizziness

Since your brain will compensate for damage that occurs to the inner ear, recurring dizziness means that repeated damage is being done. Your homework is to look for what is causing the damage to reoccur. Most likely the problem is that your diet or environment or both is increasing your histamine level. This can determined with a histamine test. Have your doctor, preferably one specializing in human biochemistry or nutrition contact a laboratory specializing in histamine testing (see chapter 13). Histamine testing may also be in order if your symptoms include itchy skin, nervous energy, hyperventilation, occasional very low energy or exhaustion. If it's determined that you do have a high histamine level, speak to your doctor about trying the diet and supplements discussed in chapters 14 and 15.

Whether you have high histamine or not you need to do some detective work to find out what is making you dizzy. If you can find the cause, you may not need to consider trying the diet and supplements discussed in this book. Finding the cause is best done by creating a diary of what you eat, drink and how you feel. If you are really thorough you might also include the pollen count, predominant pollen composition (ragweed, grass, tree, etc.), air quality, and your location (which may have dust, mold, chemicals, etc.). You need to keep recording all this information until you have had many dizziness attacks. After you have collected a good amount of data you can then look for trends. You might discover that two days before most dizziness attacks you had spaghetti or that you always feel worse when the tree pollen level is high for two or three days in a row. If you keep a very good diary, the odds that you will find out what is causing or contributing to your dizziness will be greatly increased.

See an Allergist

An additional step might be to see an allergist, especially if you think you have found a link to pollen or your environment. They can give you a Scratch or RAST allergy test (described in chapter 5) to discover if you have an allergy causing or aggravating your condition. Unfortunately, if you have a pet, it may be making your condition worse even if you're not allergic to it in a typical sense. Dog and cat dander as well as all the other "junk" your pet brings into the house on their fur may increase your histamine level. The research that you do (above) to determine the cause of your dizziness may help to better guide the allergist as to what compounds to test you for.

Chapter 20: Finding Doctors and Nutritionists

One of the best things you can do for your balance disorder is to find good doctors. The best way is to find a person locally who has the same condition as you and ask who they see. The second best method is to ask a doctor you know and trust to give you a referral. A third method is to contact the biggest, most prestigious hospital in your area and ask them for a referral. Most hospitals have nurses you can speak with who will make a recommendation among the doctors affiliated with the hospital. You can find a nutritionist the same way. Just make sure they specialize in nutrition and biochemistry. Don't be afraid to find another doctor or nutritionist if you feel they are not taking you down the right path. Unfortunately you also need to make sure that the doctor you found accepts your insurance.

Chapter 21: Benign Paroxysmal Positional Vertigo (BPPV)

Diagnosis

The simplest method to diagnose BPPV is just to tell your doctor what makes you dizzy such as tilting your head back or to the right. Unfortunately, he'll want to confirm this by having you perform these motions and watching your eye movement to make sure you are experiencing dizziness only in those positions.

BPPV can also be diagnosed using the Dix-Hallpike test. The test is performed sitting down with your legs extended. You turn your head to one side and lie down on your back quickly with your head hanging off the table. Your eyes are observed for the back and forth motion called nystagmus that occurs whenever you are dizzy. Eye movement may also be tracked and graphed using electrodes places on the head or by using a visor that monitors eye movement using an infrared camera. The side of your head that your eyes move to the fastest is the side with BPPV. The test is repeated with your head turned the other way. It is not a pleasant test.

Treating BPPV

The best method to treat BPPV is to undergo one of the two Canalith repositioning maneuvers detailed below. The maneuvers work by orienting your head in various ways to try and reposition the detached Otoconia in the inner ear to a place where it won't generate false motion signals. Both methods can cause extreme dizziness when they performed the first time, so it's recommended that they be performed by a doctor or trained vestibular therapist. After the maneuvers are completed there is a very good chance that your BPPV will be "cured".

Epley Maneuver

The Epley maneuver (name after Dr. John Epley) is used to treat BPPV and works (like the Dix-Hallpike test) by orienting your head in various ways to try and reposition the detached Otoconia in the inner ear to a place where it won't generate false motion signals. The maneuver can be done at a doctor's office, vestibular therapy center or even at home. However, I would not recommend trying it home the first time as the dizziness it causes may be so profound you may not be able to endure the process without help.

How to perform the maneuver is shown below. These steps are based on instructions posted on the Internet by Northwestern University, Copyright 1998. The instructions and photos below are my original material.

Warning:

This maneuver may cause mild to profound dizziness, usually profound the first time it's done. As I mentioned in the Preface, it felt like being thrown off a cliff. If done at home, its best done on a bed that slants back toward the head somewhat. Take precautions against falling off the bed, bumping your head, etc. It's best to have someone with you to hold your head (to reduce the sense of panic when the dizziness caused by the maneuver occurs) as well as track the time you need to remain in each position.

Important Note:

When your head is moved to any position during the maneuver that causes dizziness, the dizziness may not occur for about 15 seconds. This is because it may take some time for the Otoconia to "fall" through the liquid in the inner ear to a location that causes dizziness. This is why its import to wait at least 30 seconds before going to the next step in the maneuver.

More Important Note:

After you become (incredible) dizzy when a step in the maneuver is performed, know that if you keep your head steady in this position, the dizziness will subside to zero after 30 seconds to about two minutes. It's best to let this happen. First it will give you confidence that movements during the maneuver won't cause permanent dizziness. Second, it provides a recuperation period that will make it easier to endure the next step.

The Epley maneuver causes the most dizziness the first time it's performed. It should get easier each time it's repeated. It should be repeated until you no longer have any dizziness, although you may have to perform the maneuver for the other ear. It should only take two or three repetitions (per ear). If your dizziness if not gone by then, there may be some other issue and you should contact your doctor. However, don't be surprised if the maneuver needs to be repeated a day or two later. Hopefully, this last time maneuver will be kind of a final Otoconia "clean up" and make you much less dizzy.

Epley Maneuver Instructions

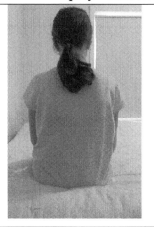

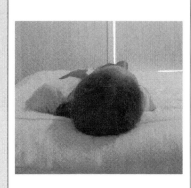

Sit upright on the bed.	Lie on your back and turn your head 45 degrees to the side causing your dizziness. Stay in this position at least 30 seconds. Hold until the dizziness subsides.

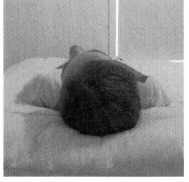

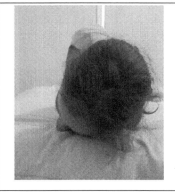

Turn your head to the opposite side at about 45 degrees. Stay in this position for at least 30 seconds. Hold until the dizziness subsides.	Roll onto your side in the same direction as the last step. Point your head so that your nose is about 45 degrees from pointing down into the bed. Stay in this position at least 30 seconds. Hold until the dizziness subsides.

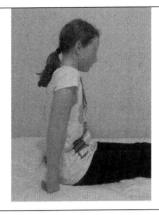

Sit up with your head tilted down for one minute or until the dizziness subsides.	Repeat the procedure two or more times until it no longer causes dizziness. It may need to be repeated for the other side (ear). Wait 10 to 15 minutes before repeating the maneuver.

Note: This maneuver may need to be repeated the next day and possibly several times a year if BPPV returns.

Half Somersault Maneuver

The Half Somersault Maneuver is a newer maneuver invented by Dr. Carol Foster. It's a Canalith Repositioning Maneuver. Like the Epley Maneuver, it's used to relocate the Otoconia in the inner ear of BPPV sufferers in order to eliminate false motion signals. I think the name of the maneuver will scare many BPPV suffers away from trying it which is unfortunate. You don't actually need to do a somersault, but just get into a tucked position as if you were going to do one. A vestibular therapist told me this maneuver worked perfectly for one of her clients who tried it at home.

Dr. Foster does not compare her maneuver to Epley, but what they try to do is identical. The Epley maneuver has a theoretical advantage in that it works within one to three repetitions where Dr. Foster recommends four to five repetitions. I believe the Half Somersault Maneuver may have an advantage in that it may be easier for some people to do at home. However, like the Epley maneuver I would not recommend trying it home the first time as the dizziness it causes may be so profound you may not be able to endure it without professional help.

If you want to try this maneuver, I suggest you go to her website for complete instructions including a demonstration video. The actual instructions start at 1:21 into the 3 minute 30 second video.

http://www.halfsomersaultmaneuver.com/video-and-step-by-step-instructions/

Chapter 22: My Life Now

After being on my diet and supplement program for a few weeks, my Meniere's symptoms, panic attacks, and most of my other symptoms began to fade; although I did have set backs from time to time.

I was on my diet and supplement program from 1995 until 2013 and after that significantly reduced my supplements, but still felt "normal" most of the time[5]. Generally, I'm not dizzy at all. I do get slightly dizzy and my ears ring a little when I cheat too much on my diet, don't take my supplements like I'm supposed to, or eat too much salt. I also tend to get a little dizzy when the air quality is poor. Poor air quality is caused by pollution trapped by stagnant air (which tends to occur on still, muggy summer days), oxygenated gasoline (used during the winter months), and during bad allergy seasons. Sometimes when I get a cold, I get dizzy for a day or so.

When I do get dizzy, it's was usually so minor that I forgot about it, especially when I'm busy. When I get a cold, sometimes the dizziness worsens, but it was still nothing compared to how dizzy I used to be and was a temporary annoyance.

I have also observed a change in my mental abilities when I'm having Meniere's symptoms. Specifically, I am more forgetful, less focused, foggy, and have more trouble doing simultaneous tasks. It's actually possible to be dizzy without feeling dizzy, which I admit is a strange concept. It seems to work like this: Something happens to

---

[5] See chapter 15, "What I take now" and chapter 24, "Postscript" for an explanation on this.

increase my histamine level (i.e. poor diet, missed supplements, too much salt, poor air quality, etc.) which causes my inner ear to transmit faulty balance signals to my brain. My brain has learned to compensate for this over time by using substitute balance signals based on my body position and vision. This compensation prevents me from feeling dizzy, but because it's causing my brain to use a lot more energy and resources to compensate, I have trouble thinking, feel foggy and am forgetful. In other words, my brain has learned to compensate for my balance problem at times by trading dizziness for fogginess and memory. These symptoms typically indicate that I need to be more careful with my diet and supplements or the next step may be actual dizziness. Fortunately, periods like this are rare and kept to a minimum through better attention to my diet and supplements.

Chapter 23: Directory of Balance Organizations

The following is a list of organizations where you can find more information or help for your balance disorder. The list is credited to National Institute on Deafness and Other Communication Disorders, National Institutes of Health so it contains many hearing references. (www.nidcd.nih.gov/health/balance/pages/balance_disorders.aspx).

Association of Late-Deafened Adults (ALDA)
Address: 8038 Macintosh Lane, Rockford, IL, 61107
E-mail: info@alda.org
Internet: www.alda.org

American Otological Society (AOS)
Address: Administrative Office, 3096 Riverdale Road, The Villages, FL, 32162
E-mail: segossard@aol.com
Internet: www.americanotologicalsociety.org

American Tinnitus Association (ATA)
Address: P.O. Box 5, Portland, OR, 97207-0005
E-mail: jennifer@ata.org
Internet: www.ata.org

American Academy of Otolaryngology--Head and Neck Surgery (AAO-HNS)
Address: 1650 Diagonal Road, Alexandria, VA, 22314-2857
E-mail: webmaster@entnet.org
Internet: www.entnet.org

American Neurotology Society (ANS)
Address: Administrative Office, 1980 Warson Road, Springfield, IL, 62704
E-mail: neurotology65@yahoo.com
Internet: www.americanneurotologysociety.com

House Research Institute
Address: 2100 West Third Street, Los Angeles, CA, 90057
E-mail: webmaster@hei.org
Internet: www.hei.org

Hearing Health Foundation
Address: 363 Seventh Avenue, 10th Floor, New York, NY, 10001-3904
E-mail: info@hearinghealthfoundation.org
Internet: hearinghealthfoundation.org

Hearing Loss Association of America
Address: 7910 Woodmont Avenue, Suite 1200, Bethesda, MD, 20814
E-mail: info@hearingloss.org
Internet: www.hearingloss.org

National Institute on Deafness and Other Communication Disorders (NIDCD)
Address: Office of Health Communication and Public Liaison, 31 Center Drive, MSC 2320, Bethesda, MD, 20892-2320
E-mail: nidcdinfo@nidcd.nih.gov
Internet: www.nidcd.nih.gov / www.noisyplanet.nidcd.nih.gov

National Organization for Rare Disorders (NORD)
Address: P.O. Box 1968, 55 Kenosia Avenue, Danbury, CT, 06813-1968
E-mail: orphan@rarediseases.org
Internet: www.rarediseases.org

National Organization for Hearing Research Foundation (NOHR)
Address: 225 Haverford Avenue, Suite 1, Narberth, PA, 19072-2234
E-mail: smsnohr@att.net
Internet: www.nohrfoundation.org

National Institute on Deafness and Other Communication Disorders
(NIDCD) Information Clearinghouse
Address: 1 Communication Avenue, Bethesda, MD, 20892-3456
E-mail: nidcdinfo@nidcd.nih.gov
Internet: www.nidcd.nih.gov

National Temporal Bone, Hearing, and Balance Pathology Resource
Registry
Address: Massachusetts Eye and Ear Infirmary, 243 Charles Street,
Boston, MA, 02114-3096
E-mail: tbregistry@meei.harvard.edu
Internet: www.tbregistry.org

St. Joseph Institute for the Deaf (SJI)
Address: 1809 Clarkson Road, Chesterfield, MO, 63017
E-mail: info@sjid.org
Internet: www.sjid.org

Vestibular Disorders Association (VEDA)
Address: P.O. Box 13305, Portland, OR, 97213-0305
Years ago refused to show a listing for this book, but now accepts paid
advertisements.
E-mail: info@vestibular.org
Internet: www.vestibular.org

Virginia Merrill Bloedel Hearing Research Center (VMBHRC)
Address: University of Washington, Box 357923, Seattle, WA, 98195-
7923
E-mail: bloedel@uw.edu
Internet: depts.washington.edu/hearing

Chapter 24: PostScript

After almost 20 years of nearly perfect blood tests, I was diagnosed several years ago with Drug Induced Hepatitis. Hepatitis is damage to the liver and it can become very serious or fatal if not treated. My tests indicated there was liver damage, but it ruled out Hepatitis A, B and C. Since I don't take drugs, my doctor attributed the Hepatitis to the either the supplements I've been taking or to blood pressure medication I had very recently started. I immediately stopped taking all supplements and the medication and after a few weeks my liver function returned to normal again.

It was eventually confirmed by the FDA, that some of the supplements I was taking manufactured by Mira Health Products Ltd. contained steroids. Apparently it took quite a bit of persuasion for the FDA to finally investigate this issue despite there being many people affected. How the steroids suddenly got into the supplements was unknown and not investigated. See the following link:

http://www.fda.gov/Safety/MedWatch/SafetyInformation/SafetyAlertsfor HumanMedicalProducts/ucm362800.htm

Supplement manufacturers are not well regulated by the FDA and apparently do not need any specific amount of insurance to compensate victims should anything "bad" occur. Strangely, even if they have insurance, they are allowed to use it for their own attorney's fees, defending the owners and company and leaving little or nothing for victims. Be very cautious about taking any supplement no matter how benign it might appear and report any changes in your health such as dark urine (a sign of liver failure) to your doctor immediately.

Questions:

info@conquer-your-balance-disorder.com

21175986R00066

Made in the USA
San Bernardino, CA
02 January 2019